PUBLIC HEALTH IN THE 21ST CENTURY

OBESITY AMONG AMERICAN INDIANS AND ALASKA NATIVES

PUBLIC HEALTH IN THE 21ST CENTURY

Additional books in this series can be found on Nova's website under the Series tab.

Additional e-books in this series can be found on Nova's website under the e-book tab.

PUBLIC HEALTH IN THE 21ST CENTURY

OBESITY AMONG AMERICAN INDIANS AND ALASKA NATIVES

TAYLOR PLASKETT
EDITOR

nova publishers
New York

Library of Congress Cataloging-in-Publication Data

ISBN: 978-1-63463-486-1

Published by Nova Science Publishers, Inc. † New York

CONTENTS

PREFACE

The book is organized into four major sections: a literature review that synthesizes research findings pertaining to the prevalence of obesity and examines what is known about the major determinants and consequences of obesity as well as the nature and findings of various types of clinical and community-based interventions; activities of selected federal agencies in the area of obesity and AI/ANs; summary of a site visit to the Gila River Indian Community; and directions for future research.

Chapter 1 – The prevalence of obesity in American Indian/Alaska Native (AI/AN) populations has increased dramatically over the past 30 years. Although AIs are not a homogeneous group, all tribes throughout the U.S. have suffered adverse effects from the high prevalence of obesity). Overall, studies demonstrate that obesity begins early for AI/AN children and also is a significant problem for the adult population. Many chronic diseases such as type 2 diabetes, heart disease, stroke, arthritis, and breathing problems are associated with the increasing prevalence of obesity in AIs.

Chapter 2 – The health risks associated with obesity make reducing the high prevalence of obesity a public health priority. Previous publications have shown both racial and ethnic disparities in obesity prevalence and no change in the prevalence of obesity among adults since 2003–2004. National obesity prevalence estimates for non-Hispanic Asian persons are possible for the first time, using newly available data. This report presents national estimates of obesity among adults in the United States in 2011–2012, based on measured weight and height.

In: Obesity Among American Indians … ISBN: 978-1-63463-486-1
Editor: Taylor Plaskett

Chapter 1

OBESITY AND AMERICAN INDIANS/ALASKA NATIVES*

Peggy Halpern

EXECUTIVE SUMMARY

Introduction

The prevalence of obesity in American Indian/Alaska Native (AI/AN) populations has increased dramatically over the past 30 years. Although AIs are not a homogeneous group, all tribes throughout the U.S. have suffered adverse effects from the high prevalence of obesity (Story et al., 2000)). Overall, studies demonstrate that obesity begins early for AI/AN children and also is a significant problem for the adult population (IHS, 2001). Many chronic diseases such as type 2 diabetes, heart disease, stroke, arthritis, and breathing problems are associated with the increasing prevalence of obesity in AIs (DHHS, 2001, Story et al., 1999).

The problem of obesity is not unique to AI/ANs. Overweight and obesity have reached epidemic proportions both nationwide and globally (Ogden et al., 2006; Washington, Post, 2006). The existence of these epidemics indicate that in addition to personal responsibility, societal factors such as convenience technology and engineering; food production and marketing patterns; and

* This is an edited, reformatted and augmented version of a report issued by the U.S. Department of Health and Human Services, April 2007.

powerful social and cultural forces that have shaped our communities, our lifestyles and ultimately our bodies play an important role in this problem (McGinnis, 2004).

The purpose of this study is to provide information that will help to understand the high rates of obesity among the AI/ANs, the nature of a variety of preventive interventions and their efficacy, and directions for future research that may involve research collaborations among government agencies and other organizations.

The report is organized into four major sections: 1) a literature review that synthesizes research findings pertaining to the prevalence of obesity and examines what is known about the major determinants and consequences of obesity as well as the nature and findings of various types of clinical and community-based interventions; 2) activities of selected federal agencies in the area of obesity and AI/ANs; 3) summary of a site visit to the Gila River Indian Community; and 4) directions for future research.

I. Literature Review

Prevalence

Available data indicate that the prevalence of overweight and obesity in AI/AN preschoolers, school-aged children and adults is higher than the respective U.S. rates for all races combined (Zephier et al., 2006; Denny et al., 2003; CDC, 2005), and trends over long periods of time indicate increasing rates of overweight and obesity for both school-aged children and adults (Zephier, 2006; White et al., 1997). Although the precise time period is not yet clear, obesity in AI/AN children generally begins in early childhood, in the preschool years. While breastfeeding may be protective against obesity in AI/ANs (Thomas & Cook, 2005), factors that contribute to the problem include prepregnancy and gestational diabetes, the weight of the mother, and childhood obesity (Salbe et al., 2000; Moum et al., 2004; Gallaher et al., 1991).

Studies have found regional and tribal variation in prevalence rates for both school-aged children and adults (Caballero et al., 2003; Denny et al., 2003). Findings on prevalence of obesity for school-aged children by gender are mixed and vary by age (Eisenmann et al., 2003; Zephier, 1999, 206; Caballero et al., 2003). For adults, some studies indicate higher prevalence of obesity/overweight in women, while other studies show no difference, and this prevalence may also vary by age (Gray et al., 2000; Giuliano et al., 1998).

Although 64 percent of AI/ANs live in urban areas, many of the prevalence studies do not include them (U.S. Census, 2006).

Contributing Factors

Nutrition and Diet. The shift in Indian Country from traditional occupations such as hunting, gathering and farming to a cash economy occurred in the early 1900's and forced family members to leave home in search of paid employment (Michel, 2004). As a result, the amount of wild and homegrown foods in the AI/AN diet has diminished, and a greater proportion of food is processed and commercially prepared, a trend also seen among the whole U.S. population. Diets historically high in complex carbohydrate/high fiber foods and lower in fat have been replaced by foods high in refined carbohydrates (e.g. refined sugars), fat, sodium, and low in fruits and vegetables (IHS, 2001). In a review of several reservation-based studies, Story et al. (2000) found that current dietary fat intake was above the Recommended Dietary Allowances (RDA) of 30 percent of total calories, ranging from 31-47 percent.

High rates of poverty (23 percent in 2001-2003) and unemployment limit access to purchased sources of a healthy food supply and promote reliance on special federal commodity programs for Indian tribes (PRC, 2004). Tribal administrators of the commodity programs have noticed improvements in the content, quality, and variety of foods offered, but say that the ingredients of the products could still be made healthier (Finegold, 2005). Pareo-Tubbeh et al. (2000) explored the variety, affordability and availability of healthful foods at convenience stores and trading posts on the Navajo Reservation. They found that while there were improvements in the availability of healthful foods from previous studies, a limited number of such foods were available at the local trading posts that are the primary, and in many cases, the only readily accessible sources of purchased food.

Socioeconomic Factors. Kumanyika and Grier (2006) review evidence that indicate the higher rates of obesity in racial and ethnic minority and low income communities are associated with a plethora of unfavorable influences – economic stresses, reduced access to affordable healthful foods, opportunities for safe and varied physical activity, overexposure to targeted advertising, and marketing of energy-dense foods.

AI/ANs face these types of socioeconomic circumstances which affect their general living conditions, their ability to find employment, the types of foods they are able to purchase, resources available for exercise and recreational activities, and overall physical and emotional health. While the circumstances of each tribe are unique, most tribes have experienced economic, education, housing, health and other problems at levels of severity rarely seen in most other American communities (Hillabrant et al., 2001).

Psychosocial Factors. Historical trauma and grief are sometimes cited as factors impacting psychological and physical health and contributing to the health disparities between AI/ANs and other groups. Historical trauma refers to the collective emotional and psychological injury both over the life span and across generations resulting from the history of difficulties that Native Americans as a group have experienced in America (Steinman, 2005). Furthermore, Brave Heart and DeBruyn (1998) point out that understanding historical trauma also involves keeping in mind the actual day-to-day traumatic losses experienced by many AI/ANs. These loses involve interpersonal, non-interpersonal and witnessed traumas such as alcohol-related accidents, homicide, and suicide.

An additional psychosocial factor that has not been carefully examined is AI/ANs perception of obesity/overweight as a problem. Some studies (White et al., 1997; Teufel & Dufour, 1990; Kumanyika, 1995) as well as anecdotal comments from Gila River Indian Community members indicate that AI/ANs view overweight/obesity as normal and healthy. Finally, while depression has not been examined in studies pertaining to AI/ANs and obesity, a few studies have found that being AI increases the likelihood of posttraumatic stress disorder (Arehart-Treichel, 2006) or of having a major depressive disorder (Hasin et al., 2006); additional research is required to determine if these conditions are associated with obesity/overweight. The relationship between obesity and depression may involve both cause and effect; while depression may be a contributor to obesity, it can also be a consequence of obesity in both adults and children (Daniels, 2006).

Genetic Factors. The role of genetics in relation to the environment is complex and is an issue where there is some disagreement. Ravussin (1995) explains that when whole populations are studied, the prevalence of obesity appears to be largely determined by environment (e.g., the Mexican Pimas compared to the Arizona Pimas), but among individuals within a given environment, variability in body size is largely influenced by genes. However, research evidence on the whole appears mixed regarding genetic factors in relation to obesity in AI/ANs. Story et al. (2003) noted that there was little evidence to support a role of energy expenditure in the development of childhood obesity, as neither energy expenditure or metabolic rate is significantly different between AI or White children; however, other researchers have identified three metabolic predictors of obesity in Pima

Indians, a group with a very high prevalence obesity and diabetes (Walston et al., 1995; Ravussin, 1995). Several researchers (Ravussin, 1995; Story et al., 2003; Harrison & Ritenbaugh, 1992) have pointed out that genetic and environmental factors may interact in AI/ANs. The environment plays a role either by compounding a genetic tendency toward weight gain or by mitigating it.

Physical Activity. Physical activity is protective against obesity and other health risks, but in the process of acculturation, AI/ANs have shifted from a traditional subsistence lifestyle to a more sedentary one that involves much less physical activity (Mendlein et al., 1997; Sugarman, 1992). Several studies (Mendlein et al., 1997; Yurgalevitch et al., 1998) have found low physical activity levels among those living in reservation-based communities as well as AI/AN urban youth (Gray and Smith, 2003). These studies suggested that environmental interventions are needed to increase opportunities for physical activity and to address barriers on reservations; for example, family-oriented physical activities or child care to allow adults with children to exercise, community centers, outdoor walking trails, and school gymnasiums open for community use (Harnack et al., 1999). And, in a school-based obesity prevention intervention with AI/ANs, Thompson et al. (2001) found a lack of facilities, equipment and trained physical education staff and before or after class activities held at the school.

Consequences of Obesity

Physical Health Consequences. Known obesity-related health risks for AI/NA adults include increased likelihood of type 2 diabetes, hypertension, cardiovascular disease (CVD), and problems with lipid levels (NRCCDH, 1989). There has been a recent significant increase in prevalence of type 2 diabetes among U.S. AI youth; this condition is now commonly seen in AI children aged 10 and over (Dabelea et al., 1998; Fagot-Campagna et al., 2000). Furthermore, childhood overweight increases the risk of adult overweight, the clustering of other CVD risk factors, coronary calcification in adulthood, and all cause CVD mortality (Power et al., 1997).

Psychosocial Consequences. Overweight and obese individuals may suffer from social stigmatization, discrimination and poor body image (U.S. DHHS, 2001; Strauss & Pollack, 2006). It is believed that these psychosocial consequences result from societal value placed on thinness as the ideal body form. However, the majority of studies in this area have been done with White populations; thus, it is unclear whether and to what degree there may be adverse psychosocial effects related to obesity in AI adults or youth (Story, 2003).

Research findings pertaining to AI/ANs indicate that adults and children understand that obesity, diabetes, heart disease and hypertension are related to dietary behavior and that physical exercise is valuable (Harnack et al., 1995; Sherwood et al., 2000; Rinderknecht & Smith, 2002). Additionally, AI children and adults are concerned about their weight, are dissatisfied with being overweight, and engage in practices to lose weight, particularly those who are overweight (Harnack et al., 1999; Story et al., 2001). However, Neumark-Sztainer et al. (1997) found that among AI youth, overweight status is not consistently associated with suicidal ideation or future job or peer concerns suggesting either greater social acceptance of overweight in the AI/AN culture or at least that overweight has a limited impact on psychosocial health. Finally, in studies involving both adults and children, some AIs were found to engage in undesirable dieting practices such as binge dieting or self-induced vomiting (Sherwood et al., 2000; Story et al., 2001).

Critical barriers to weight loss reported on in these studies included: preferences for high fat foods and their ready availability, desire for large servings, a lack of confidence for personal lifestyle change, a lack of skills needed to bring about this change, and a lack of social support for these efforts (Hood et al., 1997).

Economic Consequences. There is little information about the economic costs of obesity that is specific to AI/ANs. However, we know that obesity and overweight among all Americans are associated with both direct (e.g., preventive, diagnostic and treatment services) and indirect costs (e.g., value of lost wages). Most of these costs are due to type 2 diabetes, coronary heart disease and hypertension (Wolf & Colditz, 1998; Wolf, 2001; Wolf, 1998).

Intervention Research

Intervention research in the area of obesity prevention is in its infancy; there are only a limited number of published studies pertaining to AI/ANs. All of the interventions reviewed were implemented using Native American culture and traditions. A clinical intervention study of major importance was the *Diabetes Prevention Program (DPP)* that included AI/ANs, but was not limited to them. This study found that the Lifestyle Balance intervention was significantly more effective in reducing the incidence of diabetes and resulted in greater weight loss and increase in leisure physical activity than the placebo or the drug metformin (DDP Research Group, 2000a).

Several of the AI/AN school and/or community-based approaches reviewed did not find significant changes in youth overweight/obesity (Hood et al., 1997; Paradis et al., 2005; Davis et al., 2003). However, findings from these studies did indicate changes in mediating variables involving knowledge, attitudes or behaviors such as: increase in healthy food choices at school, additional classroom diabetes-prevention activities, positive changes in the school nutrition policy, addition of community walking paths, changes in high calorie beverage consumption, increased physical activity while at school, or reduced TV watching.

In both the clinical and community-based intervention studies that were reviewed, key Native values, culture and traditions were creatively incorporated as part of the interventions. These interventions (described in this report) have utilized various means to do this; for example, through the use of traditional Talking Circles; indigenous peer educators; community coalitions; culturally integrated curricula; or the use of traditional stories, games, music artwork, foods, or family activities.

Several emerging trends were apparent in reviewing intervention studies *currently* being implemented by federal agencies, although many of these projects have not yet completed a formal evaluation. First, in addition to behavioral approaches, several studies have focused on environmental interventions (i.e., walking trails, diet sodas in vending machines, etc.). Next, many current studies are multi-level and/or multi-component interventions that involve more than one level of the social-ecological model (i.e., community, school, individual, family) as well as more than one key strategy (i.e., physical activity, nutrition education, breastfeeding). And, finally, approaches for urban Indian women need to be less traditional than those for persons living on reservations and must adapt to the current social realities of these women.

II. Federal Agency Activities

Indian Health Service (IHS). IHS has an internal obesity workgroup that has delineated goals and action steps to address this issue. Selected activities of IHS pertaining to obesity prevention include:

- *Special Diabetes Program for Indians (SDPI).* This Congressionally-established program has funded approximately 399 grants in 35 states focusing on the prevention and treatment of diabetes in AI/ANs. It includes 66 *competitive Targeted Demonstration Projects* focusing on primary prevention of type 2 diabetes and CVD risk reduction.

- *IHS Obesity Data.* IHS uses a Resource and Patient Management System (RPMS) clinical software application called the Clinical Reporting System for national reporting and local and Area monitoring of Government Performance Results Act (GPRA) clinical performance measures, including measures pertaining to obesity.
- *On the T.R.A.I.L. (Together Raising Awareness for Indian Life) to Diabetes Prevention.* IHS, the National Congress of American Indians, Boys and Girls Clubs, Nike, and FirstPic Inc. collaborate in conducting this diabetes prevention program that takes place at Boys and Girls Clubs located in 40 Native American communities.
- *Bodyworks.* The IHS Division of Diabetes Treatment and Prevention and the Office of Women's Health (DHHS) have adapted a Bodyworks toolkit that is used in group sessions with AI/AN mothers and adolescent girls for the purpose of obesity prevention.

National Institutes of Health. The NIH supports a broad spectrum of obesity-related research and established an Obesity Research Task Force in 2003. Selected initiatives pertaining to obesity prevention include the following:

- *The Diabetes Prevention Program (DPP)* funded by the National Institute of Diabetes, Digestive and Kidney Diseases (NIDDK) (completed in 2001) and its follow-up study, the *Diabetes Prevention Program Outcomes Study* (DPPOS), that examines the long term effect of various interventions, are clinical intervention studies that include AI/ANs (in addition to other groups) and examine treatment effects by race.
- *Sharing Wisdom*, a randomized controlled trial conducted to test a lifestyle educational intervention for non-diabetic urban-dwelling AI women funded by NIDDK.
- *Diabetes Education in Tribal Schools (DETS) Program.* Tribal colleges and universities are developing a K-12 diabetes-science prevention curriculum for AI/AN students. NIDDK is lead agency collaborating with IHS and CDC.
- *National Diabetes Education Program (NDEP).* This public awareness and education campaign is sponsored by NIDDK and CDC and has a specialized component that tailors messages to AI/ANs.

- *Community-Responsive Interventions to Reduce Cardiovascular Risk in AI/ANs.* The National Heart Lung and Blood Institute (NHLBI) has initiated cooperative agreements in AI/AN communities for the purpose of testing the effectiveness of behavioral and/or environmental interventions to promote the adoption of healthy lifestyles.

Centers for Disease Control and Prevention (CDC). Selected activities pertaining to obesity prevention include:

- *Native Diabetes Wellness program (NDWP).* The Division of Diabetes Translation sponsors the NDWP, a collaboration with IHS that sponsors various activities including the DETS Program (noted above). Additionally, cooperative agreements have been awarded to tribal communities for the purpose of testing community environmental adaptations for diabetes prevention.
- *PedNSS and PNSS.* The Division of Nutrition and Physical Activity operate the Pediatric Nutrition surveillance System (PedNSS) and the Pregnancy Nutrition Surveillance System (PNSS), program-based systems that monitor the nutritional status of low-income infants, children and women in federally funded programs, including AI/ANs.
- *Well-Integrated Screening and Evaluation for Women Across the Nation (WISEWOMAN) Program.* The Division for Heart Disease and Stroke Prevention funds this screening and lifestyle intervention program for low income women that addresses risk factors for heart disease including obesity and includes two programs serving ANs.

United States Department of Agriculture (USDA). Selected activities of USDA include:

- *National Research Initiative: Human Nutrition and Obesity.* The USDA has a cross- cutting competitive grant program that funds research projects pertaining to various topic areas including obesity prevention with a focus on populations at risk; for example, the *Seven Generations of Health: A Transgenerational Approach to Human Nutrition and Obesity Intervention in Indian Country* was funded. The purpose of this project is to disseminate culturally relevant information about obesity prevention in Indian Country and to establish a community-based infrastructure for healthy lifestyles in four Native American communities that reflects differing generations.

- *Food Distribution Program on Indian Reservations (FDPIR).* FDPIR provides commodity foods (e.g., canned vegetables, cereal, evaporated milk, fruit juice) to low income households located on Indian reservations.

III. Site Visit to Gila River Indian Community

This section of the report includes information gathered during a site visit to the Gila River Indian Community of the Gila River Indian Reservation (40 miles south of Phoenix) in January 2006. The community is composed of members of the Pima and Maricopa Tribes. The purpose of this visit was to learn about obesity treatment and prevention activities. Interviews were held with staff from the Health Corporation, the tribe's Department of Human Resources and the National Institute of Diabetes and Digestive and Kidney Diseases (NIDDK) researchers based in Phoenix. The site visit report covers: background information, food availability, recreational facilities, attitudes about obesity, psychosocial issues, intervention programs, and NIDDK research studies conducted with this tribe.

IV. Directions for Future Research

Additional studies that are specific to AI/AN and obesity are needed in many areas. A list of these areas along with some key knowledge gaps follows:

- *Prevalence.* Longitudinal studies are needed to determine growth patterns over time so that critical intervention points can be identified. Factors contributing to regional differences in obesity rates also need to be examined. Further study can explore the prevalence of obesity in AI/ANs living in urban areas. Improved surveillance systems need to be established so that data can be shared with tribal communities.
- *Nutrition and Diet.* Studies that examine how USDA's Food and Nutrition service can most effectively deliver nutrition education to the tribes would be useful. Among those AI/ANs who are the consumers of the Food Stamp and FDPIR programs, the question of

why the participation rate in the FDPIR program has decreased in recent years needs exploration. Studies of nutrition and physical activity patterns among AI/AN children may be useful in terms of learning more about obesity prevention.

- *Psychosocial Factors.* Studies that examine obesity in terms of its relationship to stress, mental illness and depression, psychosocial factors, environmental factors, and attitudes about obesity in AI/ANs are needed.
- *Genetics.* Continued research is needed to examine the interactions between genetic and environmental factors in the AI/AN population.
- *Intervention Research.* Intervention research can be used to explore a variety of questions such as: 1) How can intervention programs successfully address constraints to program participation?; 2) What AI/AN at-risk groups should be targeted for early intervention to prevent obesity?; 3) What family processes and behaviors contribute to obesity?; 4) What are the key mediating variables that need to be addressed in community and school-based interventions?; 5) What type of interventions focusing on the macro- environment have had successful outcomes?; and 6) How can participatory research be used to study obesity prevention in AI/AN communities?

References

The references used in the Executive Summary are located in the corresponding reference sections of the main sections of this report.

I. Literature Review

Introduction

Background

The prevalence of obesity in American Indian/Alaska Native (AI/AN) population has increased dramatically over the past 30 years. Although AIs are not a homogeneous group, all tribes have suffered adverse effects from the high prevalence of obesity (Story et al., 2000). Overall, studies demonstrate that obesity begins early for AI/AN children and also is a significant problem for the adult population (IHS, 2001). Many chronic diseases such as type 2 diabetes, heart disease, stroke, arthritis, breathing problems and psychological disorders such as depression are associated with the increasing prevalence of obesity in AIs (DHHS, 2001b; Story et al., 1999). Intervention research is needed in AI/AN communities to develop and test effective strategies for obesity prevention and treatment (Story et al., 2003).

The problem of obesity is not unique to AI/ANs. Overweight and obesity have reached epidemic proportions both nationally and globally (Ogden, 2006; Washington Post, 2006). Almost two- thirds of American adults are overweight, up from 46 percent in 1980. Of these, almost one-third are obese, meaning they weight about 30 pounds more than they should. That's a doubling in the obesity rates over 20 years (McGinnis, 2004). Furthermore, over the past three decades, the share of children who are considered overweight *or* obese has doubled from 15 percent in the 1970's to nearly 30 percent today, while the percentage of obese youth aged 12-19 has doubled (from 6.1 percent to 15.5 percent) and more than tripled for children aged 6-11 years (from 4 percent to 15.3 percent) (Koplan et al., 2005). In 2004, the Institute of Medicine released a report calling the prevention of childhood obesity a national priority (Paxson et al., 2006). In early 2000, the release of Healthy People 2010 identified overweight and obesity as major public health problems and set national objectives for reduction in their prevalence (DHHS, 2001a).

Many factors contribute to the obesity epidemic. In addition to personal responsibility, societal factors such as convenience technology and engineering; food production and marketing patterns; and powerful social and cultural forces that have shaped our communities, our lifestyles and ultimately our bodies play an important role in this problem (McGinnis, 2004).

Purpose of Study

The purpose of this study is to provide information that will help to understand the high rates of obesity among the AI/ANs, the nature of a variety of preventive interventions and their efficacy, and directions for future research that could involve research collaborations among government agencies and other organizations. The key research questions that this literature review addresses are:

- *Prevalence.* What data are available and what do we know about the prevalence of obesity in the AI/AN population, including adults, children and adolescents? Does prevalence differ by gender? How has prevalence changed over time? How does prevalence vary by tribe and by region?

- *Consequences.* What data are available with regard to the health, psychosocial and economic consequences of obesity for AI/ANs?
- *Contributing Factors.* What are the primary contributing factors pertaining to obesity in the AI/AN population? What is the role of socioeconomic factors, reservation/urban residence, genetics, lifestyle (e.g., diet/nutrition, physical activity), environment, culture, and mainstream societal factors? What is the relationship between these factors and tribe/region?
- *Interventions.* What intervention studies have been conducted, and how are outcomes being measured? What type of preventive interventions have been implemented (families, schools, communities, health care settings), and what do we know about the strategies utilized in these programs? What activities is the federal government currently implementing or planning in this area?
- *Directions for Future Research.* Where are the research and evaluation gaps, and what are the key directions for future research?

This report reviews a sample of the available research literature pertaining to obesity and AI/ANs. While the primary focus of this report is on obesity and obesity prevention, there is an unavoidable overlap with some literature pertaining to both diabetes and cardiovascular disease (CVD) because the prevention of both of these conditions involves targeting overweight and/or obesity. Thus, some studies pertaining to diabetes and CVD prevention are included in this review.

There is limited research information about obesity and Alaska Natives (ANs). Most AN villages are composed of fewer than 500 people. The remoteness, geographical barriers, cultural diversity, and roadless nature of rural Alaska presents researchers with significant logistical challenges that increase the costs of conducting studies with AN communities (Boyer et al., 2005). Likewise, there is a paucity of research pertaining to obesity and urban Indians, even though two-thirds of AI/ANs live in urban areas rather than on or near reservations. In 2000, about 34 percent of the AI/AN population lived on or near reservations, 2 percent lived in Alaska Native Village Statistical Areas, and 64.1 percent lived outside these tribal areas (U.S. Census, 2000). Whenever research pertaining to urban Indians was located, it was included in this report.

Obesity is a multifaceted topic that cuts across various dimensions of health and human services. DHHS' Office of the Assistant Secretary for Planning and Evaluation has an integrated research agenda pertaining to AI/ANs that focuses on both health and human service issues. Thus, this report is a result of collaboration between ASPE's Office of Health Policy and its Office of Human Services policy.

This report has four major sections:

- The first section is a literature review that synthesizes key themes pertaining to the prevalence of obesity in AI/AN children and adults and examines what is known about the major determinants and consequences of obesity. Studies pertaining to various types of interventions are also reviewed.
- The second section samples some of the key activities and research being conducted by four federal agencies B IHS, NIH, CDC, and USDA.
- The third section describes a site visit to the Gila River Indian Community in order to examine the issue of obesity and relevant interventions in this tribe.
- The fourth section of the report outlines research gaps and possible directions for future research gleaned from a synthesis of the literature review and discussions with key informants from federal agencies.

Prevalence

Introduction

In examining obesity/overweight prevalence for adults and children, it is critical to understand how overweight and obesity are commonly measured. An expert panel, convened by the National Institutes of Health (NIH) in 1998 utilized Body Mass Index (BMI) for defining overweight and obesity. BMI is a measure of weight in relation to height used for adults and is calculated as weight in pounds divided by the square of the height in inches, multiplied by 703, or weight in kilograms divided by the square of the height in meters. Many organizations that have endorsed the NIH guidelines, support the use of a BMI of 30 kg/m or greater to identify obesity in adults and a BMI between 25 kg/m and 29.9 kg/m to identify overweight in adults. These definitions are based on evidence that suggests health risks are greater at or above a BMI of 25Kg/m compared to those at a BMI below that level (DHHS, 2001).

In children and adolescents, overweight has been defined as a sex- and age-specific BMI at or above the 95th percentile, based on revised Centers for Disease Control and Prevention (CDC) growth charts. Neither a separate definition for obesity nor a definition for overweight based on health outcomes or risk factors is defined for children and adolescents (DHHS, 2001).

This section will include a separate discussion of prevalence for infants and preschool children, school-aged children and adults. Caution is urged when comparing the prevalence rates in various studies within each of these groups because the studies often use different standards (e.g., obese, overweight), different reference criteria (e.g., NHANES, CDC) from different years, and various sample sizes.

Infants and Preschool Children

Obesity in AI/AN children appears to begin in early childhood. In recent selected studies of preschool children of various ages (Table 1), AI/AN obesity prevalence rates are higher than similar U.S. all races rates for children 0-11 months, 12-23 months, and 24-25 months.

Two important studies sampled AI/AN children from the Women Infants and Children (WIC) Program. WIC is administered by U.S. Department of Agriculture (USDA) and provides supplemental foods, nutrition education and health care referrals to pregnant and postpartum women, infants and children up to age 5. In the first of these studies, Cole (2002), found that Native American infants and children (residing both on and off reservations) had greater risk prevalence compared to all WIC infants and children in most of the major risk categories of their study including high weight-for-height and inadequate nutrient intake (N= 27,656 AI infants; 68,041 AI children; total database of 8,042,758). Additionally, there were some differences by reservation status; for example, overweight prevalence was 20 percent for Native American children living on or near reservations, 16 percent for Native American children off reservations, and 13 percent for all WIC children.

In the second study utilizing a WIC sample, *The Pediatric Height and Weight Study in AI and AN Population 2001-2004*, Mahal et al. (2006) concluded that their results clearly demonstrated the huge disparity in prevalence of *at-risk for overweight* and *overweight* in AI/AN children that live on or near reservations as compared to other racial and ethnic groups and the general population. This study analyzed data based on a random sample of 3,251 children from WIC and Head Start agencies within the 12 IHS Service Areas, excluding Alaska and the Navajo Nation. Using CDC's national standards for overweight and obesity, findings indicated that children *under 1 year* had twice the prevalence of overweight compared to CDC's Pediatric Nutrition Surveillance System (PedNSS) data (CDC, 2005) based on more than 7 million children 0-5 years in federally-funded maternal and child health programs, and *1 year old children* had 80-97 percent higher prevalence of overweight compared to the PedNSS data. Among children *age 2-4 years*, the prevalence of *at-risk for overweight* was twice as high (38.6 percent) compared to the PedNSS data (15.7 percent), and the prevalence of *overweight* of these children was 37 percent higher (20.2 percent) than the national data (14.7 percent). There was little or no difference in the prevalence of at-risk for overweight and overweight by gender.

When Mahal et al., combined at-risk for overweight and overweight prevalence, the prevalence rate of the study data was nearly twice the CDC's prevalence rate (58.8 percent versus 30.4 percent). When comparing prevalence among different non-AI/AN racial and ethnic groups, AI/AN children age 2-4 years in this study had at least 104 percent higher prevalence of *at-risk for overweight*, and the prevalence of *overweight* was at least 60 percent higher than other racial and ethnic groups, except Hispanics who had a similar rate.

One factor that may be associated with these differences is gestational diabetes. There is a high prevalence of prepregnancy and gestational diabetes among Native Americans. Moum et al. (2004) found that Montana and North Dakota Indian mothers were more likely than white mothers to have diabetes in pregnancy (Moum et al., 2004). Children of Pima Indian women who have diabetes during pregnancy are on the average larger for gestational age at birth and are more likely to become obese in childhood than the children of women without diabetes (Pettitt et al., 1993).

Childhood obesity may lead to youth or adult obesity. A study with Pima Indian children (Salbe et al., 2002) found that early childhood obesity was the most potent predictor of obesity 5 years later. Furthermore, Lindsay et al. (2002) found that Pima Indian preschoolers in Arizona between 1-6 months and 2-11 years, gained weight at a greater rate than the reference population that was drawn from five population surveys conducted in the U.S. between 1963-1994 and published by the National Center for Health Statistics. Additionally, other research has found that infants of all races who gain weight too fast between 0-4 months may be prone to obesity later in life (Stettler et al., 2002).

Table 1. Selected Studies Describing the Prevalence of Overweight in AI/AN Infants and Preschool Children

Population/Year	Age	Sample Size	Definition of Overweight	Male	Percentage Female	Both	Source
AI, National, 2004	0-11 mo	23,244	a			13.6	PedNSS, CDC (2005)
AI, National, 2004	12-23 mo	16,866	a			25.6	PedNSS, CDC (2005)
AI, National, 2004	24-59 mo	34,330	a			19.0	
AI, National, 2001-2004	0-2 years	1,448 (M) 1,312 (F)	a	24.6	22.9		Mahal (2006)
AI, National, 2001-2004	2-4 years	1,032 (M) 1,000 (F)	a	18.6	18.2		Mahal (2006)
Mohawk, NY, 2000	2-5 years	613 (M) 500 (F)	b	20.9 –3 yr 15.7 –4 yr 16.4 –5 yr	8.4 - 2 yr 9..3 - 3 yr 14.3 – 4 yr 4.7 – 5 yr		Harvey-Berino et al. (2000)
All Races, 2004	0-11 mo	2,245,268	a			11.1	PedNSS, CDC (2005)
All Races, 2004	12-23 mo	1,460,417	a			17.7	PedNSS, CDC (2005)
All Races, 2004	24-59 mo	2,766,571	a			14.8	PedNSS, CDC (2005)

a: BMI >95th percentile. Based on 2000 CDC growth chart percentiles for weight-for-length for children under 2 years and BMI-for- age for children 2 years of age and older. See www.cdc.gov/growthcharts/

b: BMI >95th percentile. Based on NHANES II.

Table 2. Selected Studies Describing the Prevalence of Overweight in AI/AN School Children

Population/Year	Age	Sample Size	Definition of Overweight	Male	Percentage Female	Both	Source
School-Aged Children							
AI, SD, ND, IO, NB, 2002-2003	5-17 years	11,538	a	29.4	26.1		Zephier et al., (2006)
AI, Hopi, 2001-2003	6-12 years	263	b	22.6	24.0	24.0	Eisenmann et al., (2003)
AI, AZ, NM, SD, 1997-2000	8-10 years	1,704	a	26.8	30.5	28.6	Caballero et al. (2003)
All Races, 1999-2000	6-11 years	1,054	a	16.0	14.5	15.3	Ogden et al., (2002)
All Races, 1999-2000	12-19 yrs	2,244	a	15.5	15.5	15.5	Ogden et al., (2002)

Definitions of Overweight:

a: BMI >95th percentile. Based on 2000 CDC growth chart percentiles for weight-for-length for children under 2 years and BMI-for- age for children 2 years of age and older. See www.cdc.gov/growthcharts/

b: Based on age- and sex-specific CDC/NCHS 5th percentiles of the BMI. Obesity = BMI > 30. International reference values developed by Childhood Obesity Working Group of International Obesity Task Force.

This period of early rapid weight gain is more common in formula fed than breastfed infants, which could explain the protective effects of breastfeeding against childhood obesity in some but not all research studies (Murphy; Thomas & Cook, 2005). Thomas and Cook (2005) found in their study (N=81) that any amount of breastfeeding may significantly reduce the number of AI/AN preschool children who are overweight or obese; for example, 21 percent of children aged 3-4 years were overweight in the breastfeeding group versus 52 percent in the formula fed group.

Because of the potential protective effect of breastfeeding on obesity noted above, it is relevant to ask how Native Americans view this practice. One study (Wright 1993) indicated that both motherhood and breastfeeding have been and are highly valued among Navajo women. Ethnographic interviews with male and female elders in this study revealed that breast milk is valued for its nutritious qualities and that breastfeeding is important because it shows the child that it is loved. Breastfed children are viewed as better able to hear traditional teachings, to be more disciplined and to live a better life. In contrast bottle fed children are thought to be unloved, to suffer an inner sense of rejection and to be more likely to engage in bad behaviors, particularly alcohol abuse.

In a study of Mescalero Apache preschool children (Gallaher et al., 1991) found that maternal obesity and high birth weight were the factors most strongly associated with childhood obesity. They found that children with obese mothers were 2.5 times more likely to be obese than children of nonobese mothers (N=261). Studies have shown that obese women tend to have children of higher birth weight, and that these children are more likely to remain taller and heavier than children of lower birth weight.

CDC's 2004 Pregnancy Nutrition Surveillance data indicates that prepregnancy overweight (i.e., BMI > 26; includes overweight and obese women) for AI/AN women is 52.2 percent compared to White, not Hispanic – 41.5 percent; Black, not Hispanic – 50.4 percent; Hispanic – 41.5 percent; Asian/Pacific Islander – 26.1 percent; and all races – 43.3 percent. Furthermore, CDC's 2004 Pediatric Nutrition Surveillance data (CDC, 2005) indicates that AI/ANs have 9.8 percent high birth weight babies (i.e. > 4000 g) compared to White, not Hispanic (7.8 percent), Black, not Hispanic (4.5 percent), Hispanic (7.2 percent), Asian/Pacific Islander (5.7 percent) and total all race/ethnic groups (6.8 percent).

Most of the studies on preschoolers concluded that primary prevention must begin early. Mahal et al. (2006) recommend that tribal and Indian Health Service (IHS) protocols should be developed and implemented to identify high-risk children, such as children of parents who are overweight, children from a diabetic pregnancy and children with a family history of diabetes, in order to provide early and intensive interventions with rigorous follow-up, including nutrition counseling focused on infant and toddler feeding practices.

School-aged Children

Studies that examine the prevalence of overweight and/or obesity in AI/ANs have found these conditions are more likely in AI/AN school children compared to all race national averages for similar aged children (Zephier et al., 1999; Caballero et al., 2003; Jackson, 1993; Eisenmann et al., 2000; Zephier et al., 2006). See Table 2 for a listing of selected group of thesc studies and their findings.

This trend is evident by the time the children reach elementary school – as early as kindergarten to 2nd grade (Caballero et al., 2003; Zephier, 2006). Recently Zephier et al. found that at 5 years of age, more than 40 percent of their sample (N=11, 538) had BMI's equal to or greater than the 85th percentile and almost one quarter of these children had BMI's equal to or exceeding the 95th percentile. These findings are important because evidence indicates that childhood overweight increases the risk of adult overweight in addition to other negative health consequences (Eisenmann et al., 2000). Additionally, these findings highlight the need to consider obesity prevention programs for preschool-aged children, in addition to programs targeting elementary schools (Caballero et al., 2003).

Furthermore, several studies have found trends indicating increasing rates of overweight and obesity among AI school children over various time periods (Eisenmann, 2000; Caballero et al., 2003; Sugarman et al., 1990; Hrdlicka, 1908; Knowler et al., 1991; et al; Zephier, 2006).

Findings on differences by sex among school-aged children vary. Some studies indicate no significant differences between the sexes with regard to obesity or overweight among Hopi or Navajo youth (Eisenmann et al., 2000, 2003). However, Zephier (1999) found that the prevalence of obesity in males exceeded that of females at many ages, while Caballero et al. (2003) found inconsistent results. They found that the overall prevalence of overweight was somewhat higher in girls than in boys (30.5% compared with 26.8%), but in some communities, this prevalence was higher in boys, and in others there was little difference between the sexes. Recently, Zephier et al. (2006) found that in the Aberdeen Indian Health Service Area, overweight and obesity were slightly greater in boys than girls until the early teen years, when the trend reversed.

Caballero et al. (2003) also found regional/tribal variation in both overweight and obesity. For example, the percentage of obese female children (BMI> 95th percentile) ranged from 23.4 percent (Navajo) to 53.5 percent (Gila River, Pima-Maricopa), and the percentage of obese male children ranged from 20.5 percent (Navajo) to 49.4 percent (Tohono O'odham). Similarly, in earlier studies (1990-1991) considerable regional variation in overweight among school children was found ranging from 25.3 percent of children in the Navajo region to 45 percent in the Phoenix and Nashville IHS regions (Broussard, 1995).

Many of these studies do not include urban Indian school children; research with this population is sparse. Smith and Rinderknecht (2003) found a high prevalence of obesity in urban AI children aged 5-18 (N=155) that paralleled that of Native youth living on reservations. Gray and Smith (2003) also found that 59 percent of the urban Indian children in their study were sedentary. Television viewing averaged 3.9 hours per day with 13-18 year old children watching the most television. These youth were from predominantly lower income families, and many lived in high crime areas. Watching TV offers safe entertainment, and parents reported that neighborhood safety as a major public health concern for their families.

Adults

In most of the studies conducted with adult AI/NAs, prevalence rates of obesity/overweight are higher than the respective U.S rates for all races combined (Story et al., 1999; Casper et al., 1996; Welty et al., 2002; and Denny et al., 2003, Sugarman et al., 1992). Selected studies pertaining to AI/AN adults are summarized in Table 3.

Liao et al. (2003) compared the self-reported health status of AIs with other racial/ethnic minority populations using data from the Racial and Ethnic Approaches to Community Health (REACH) 2010 project. The sample included 1,791 AIs, 10,953 blacks, 4,257 Hispanics, and 4,204 Asians. Results indicated that AIs had a higher prevalence of chronic disease risk factors including obesity than other racial/ethnic minority populations. Obesity rates for AI men were 40.1 percent compared to 26.5 percent, 26.6 percent and 2.7 percent for black, Hispanics and Asian men respectively. Similar rates for AI women were 37.7 percent compared to 37.6, 28.4 percent, and 3.1 percent for black, Hispanics and Asian women respectively.

Studies of Navajo adults (Hall et al., 1992; White et al., 1997) and of Pima Indians (Knowler et al., 1991) found that the prevalence of overweight has increased over a 25-40 year period. However, in the Strong Heart Study, Welty et al. (2002) found that the prevalence of obesity among 12 tribes in Arizona, Oklahoma, and North and South Dakota remained stable over several four year periods between 1989-1991 and 1993-1995, but these rates were much higher than national rates of obesity in the total adult population.

Regional and tribal variation in prevalence exists. Denny et al. (2003) reported findings from the Behavioral Risk Factor Surveillance System (BRFSS) from 1997-2000 which utilizes self-report measures. This data reveals that Alaska Natives reported the highest prevalence of obesity for both men and women compared to other regions. Obesity prevalence rates (BMI > 30) for both men and women ranged from 21.6 percent in the Pacific Coast area to 29.0 percent in Alaska. For men, the range was between 22.8 percent in the Northern Plains to 26.9 percent in Alaska, and for women obesity prevalence ranged from 20.2 percent in the Pacific Coast to 31.1 percent in Alaska. In a study specifically focusing on ANs in the Bering Strait region, Risica et al. (2000) found a pattern of upper body fatness in Eskimo women.

Table 3. Selected Studies Describing the Prevalence of Obesity in AI/AN Adults

Population/Year	Age	Sample Size	Definition of Overweight	Male	Percentage Female	Both	Source
AI, Pima, 1993-1995	45-74 yrs	1,206	a	48.3	65.0		Welty et al., (2002)
AI, OK, 1993-1995	45-74 yrs	1,255	a	49.5	54.4		Welty et al., (2002)
AI, SD/ND, 1993-1995	45-74 yrs	1,177	a	34.2	48.5		Welty et al., (2002)
AI, Montana, 1999	> 18 yrs	1,000	b	30.0	35.0		Harwell et al., (2001)
All Races, 1999-2002	≥ 20 years	4,390	c	27.6	33.2	30.4	Hedley et al., (2004)

a: Obesity defined based on revised definitions from the general US population from the NHANES III. Obesity defined as BMI > 30.

b: BMI measured by self-report of height and weight. Obesity defined as BMI > 30.0

c: Obesity defined as BMI > 30.

The Strong Heart Study (Welty et al., 2002) conducted from 1993-1995 compared tribes from Arizona, Oklahoma and South and North Dakota and also documented varying rates of obesity; for example prevalence rates for men were 48.3 percent (AZ), 49.5 percent (OK) and 34.2 percent (SD/ND) and for women were 65.0 percent, 54.4 percent, and 48.5 percent respectively. Regional variation is also evident in the FY 2004 IHS data (includes children and adults 2-74 years); for example, obesity prevalence rates by IHS area (areas not identified) range from 34.6 percent to 57.8 percent (Cullen, 2005). Because of these differences, researchers recommend that prevention programs need to focus on local communities and utilize data that is specific to these areas or tribes (Broussard et al., 1995).

Some studies have found differences in prevalence by gender; for example Broussard et al. (1995), Gray et al. (2000) and Campos-Outcalt et al. (1995) found higher rates of obesity/overweight in women versus men. However, other studies have found that prevalence rates were identical for men and women (Denny et al., 2003; Casper et al., 1996). Table 3 includes a select group of four recent adult AI samples of varying ages in different areas of the U.S.; in these studies, the AI women had a greater prevalence of obesity compared to the men.

Findings on age-related trends in obesity/overweight rates are mixed and appear to differ by gender. Several studies have found that rates increase with age for both sexes (Harwell et al., 2001) or increase up to age 65 for women (Giuliano et al., 1998) or for men up to 59 years (Gray et al., 1999), while other studies found the prevalence of obesity/overweight decreases with increasing age in men and in diabetic women (Gray et al., 1999; White et al., 1997). A few studies found no age-related trends for nondiabetic women (Gray et al., 1999; White et al., 1997).

Contributing Factors

Nutrition and Diet

Key Trends

The shift in Indian Country from traditional occupations such as hunting, gathering and farming to a cash economy occurred in the early 1900's and forced family members to leave home in search of paid employment (Michel, 2004). As a result, the amount of wild and homegrown foods in the AI/AN diet has diminished, and a greater proportion of food is processed and commercially prepared, a trend also seen among the whole U.S. population. Diets historically high in complex carbohydrate/high fiber foods have been replaced by foods high in refined carbohydrates (e.g. refined sugars), fat, sodium, and low in fruits and vegetables (IHS, 2001).

As a result of these trends, the nutritional health of AI/AN children has changed dramatically over the past 30 years. While the prevention and treatment of malnutrition was a major health issue until the mid to late 70's, increased food availability and food assistance programs and improved sanitation, transportation, and health care have reduced malnutrition as a major health issue. However, this trend has been accompanied by a rapid increase in childhood obesity among the AI/ANs (Story et al., 1998).

High rates of AI/AN poverty and unemployment in the U.S. limit access to purchased sources of a healthy food supply and promote reliance on special federal commodity programs for Indians (PRC, 2006). Today, many tribal members exist on a steady diet of government commodities (Michel, 2004), and access to healthy food in isolated areas may be difficult due to only a few grocery stores and a limited selection in these stores (Finegold, 2005). Furthermore, the recent proliferation of fast-food restaurants and convenience food stores on or near reservations encourages the consumption of high-fat, high-sugar foods (Brossard et al., 1995; Sugarman et al., 1990).

Traditional Practices and Food

Traditional foods often have spiritual and social values; for example, they represent purity, healthfulness and strength – symbols of a pre-reservation culture, in contrast to the modern day diet (Story et al., 2000). And, food is considered a gift from the creator (deGonzague, 1999). Many traditional belief systems include the concepts of harmony and balance in respect to food, and these concepts can motivate individuals and communities to increase their use of traditional foods and adopt healthier lifestyles (Story et al., 2000). Examples of these types of foods include: wild rice (Minnesota), berries, teas, blue corn (Southwest), squash, roots, beans, salmon (Pacific Northwest) and other fish, fermented foods (e.g., heads and eggs of salmon) seal, beaver, bison (Plains) caribou, deer meat, wild game, whale. Most of these traditional foods are high in protein and low in fat and sugar.

However, some studies report that traditional foods seem to be consumed only occasionally; for example on special occasions or in ceremonies (Brown & Brenton, 1994, Grant et al., 2000, Phillips & Finn, 2000). The data reflect the change from a traditional mode of obtaining food to one of buying store bought goods. Fast food restaurants and convenience stores are often utilized as places to eat, similar to off-reservation trends (Grant et al., 2000). Furthermore, the limited use of traditional foods has been accompanied by a loss of social communication and a reduction in the teaching and knowledge passed down from elders to the next generation in regard to harvesting and consumption (deGonzague et al., 1999, Phillips & Finn, 2000). However, one study reported that the extent and use of traditional foods and harvesting practices is often unrecognized or underestimated by non-Native health care providers. For example, DeGonzague et al. (1999) in their study of Ojibwe Indians found that at least 50 percent of respondents (N=104) engaged in hunting, fishing and gathering practices.

Alaska Natives are unique in their use of traditional or subsistence foods. The Alaska Traditional Diet Survey (ATDS) was conducted to identify the most commonly consumed subsistence foods among residents of villages in rural Alaska for the eventual purpose of prioritizing foods to be tested for contaminants (ANHB/ANEC, 2004). A convenience sample of 665 participants between 13-88 years of age from 13 villages (in five regional health corporations) was surveyed. Findings indicated the following food consumption patterns:

- Two thirds or more of the participants consumed several species of fish in all five regions;
- Eighty-six percent or more consumed moose and/or caribou in all regions except one where 91 percent of participants consumed deer;
- Eighty-seven percent of the participants in each region consumed two kinds of wild berries;
- Seventy-nine percent of participants in all regions except one consumed geese;
- Nearly all participants consumed substantial amounts of store foods including fruits and vegetables; and,
- Sugared beverages and soda pop were in the top four items in all regions potentially contributing to excess calories and tooth decay;

In the ATDS, traditional foods accounted for between 12-34 percent of total energy intake by region. Seventy-four percent of participants said using subsistence foods was very important to them, 13 percent said it was somewhat important, and only 13 percent said using these foods did not matter to them. Forty-seven percent said they consumed about the same amount of subsistence foods as they had 5 years ago, 27 percent said they consumed less, and 26 percent said they consumed more.

The reasons the ANs gave for eating more traditional food now than 5 years ago included the belief that these foods are healthier than store foods, preference for their taste, lower expense, and the expressly stated cultural importance of subsistence foods. The reasons given for eating less of these foods now included: not having anyone to hunt for the family, working at a job or not having time to hunt and gather, living away from the village, lack of transportation to hunt and gather, and not having the traditional knowledge to hunt and gather. However, the most common reason was a reduction in the availability or quality of fish and animals. Common concerns expressed about subsistence food were observations of fish and animals with parasites, diseases, or lesions; reduced numbers of fish and animals; and the possible presence of contaminants in fish and animals.

The researchers concluded that for ANs, harvesting and eating subsistence foods are essential to personal, social and cultural identity. Furthermore, they stated that the majority of Alaskans could not afford to replace subsistence foods with store foods. Because rural Alaskans consume large quantities of subsistence foods, there is a potential risk of their exposure to contaminants that may be in these foods. However, the data to assess exposure are inadequate because many traditional subsistence foods have not been tested.

Dietary Studies

There is a paucity of research pertaining to diet in Indian Country, and existing studies focus on reservation-based rather than urban samples. In an extensive review of the dietary literature covering 1980-1998, Story et al. (2000), examined 13 studies reporting nutrient intakes in 20 tribal groups. Sample sizes ranged from 21-946 with ages from 10-91 years. Major findings included:

- Dietary fat intake was above the Recommended Dietary Allowances (RDA) of 30 percent of total calories, ranging from 31-47 percent. A fat intake above the RDA is also a concern for the general population;
- Mean intakes of vitamin A were below the RDA for all age groups and both genders in the Navajo Health & Nutrition Survey;
- Calcium intake was below the RDA for most of the groups, and this is a concern for the general population as well;
- RDA for iron was not met for most of the groups of females, and this is a concern for the general population as well as AI/ANs;
- In all of the studies, the mean protein intake met RDAs; and
- Vitamin C intake was adequate in all groups except Cherokee boys in North Carolina.

Several later studies not included in Story's review found that AI diets were of lower quality than those of the general population. For example, deGonzague et al. (1999) in their study of two Ojibwe communities (N=104) in Minnesota and Wisconsin found that intake of fiber was lower and of fats and saturated fats was higher. Additionally, mean intakes of vitamin A and calcium were below the RDA for men and mean intakes of vitamin A, folate, calcium, iron, and zinc were below the RDA for women. They concluded that culturally relevant nutrition programs were needed and that that low fat traditional food preparation methods be promoted. Also, Phillips and Finn (2000) found in studying Cheyenne River Lakota households (N=216) that a lack of fruit and vegetable consumption reduced the intake of essential nutrients. In addition, they found that sweetened beverages were consumed at high levels.

Story et al. (2002) examined school meals served in 41 elementary schools (e.g, public, private, BIA, tribal contract schools) on 7 reservations in New Mexico, South Dakota, and Arizona. All the schools participated in the National School Lunch Program and three offered the School Breakfast Program. They found that the average elementary school lunch exceeds one-third of the recommended daily nutrient intakes for children for most nutrients, and the average school breakfast also exceeded one-fourth of the recommended intakes for all nutrients except folate. However, the average school lunch provided 33 percent of total energy from fat, which exceeded the goal of <30 percent of total energy from fat. In a recent USDA study (Fox et al., 2001), the mean percentage of energy from fat in elementary schools across the United States was also 33 percent. Story et al., also found that school breakfasts met the Dietary Guidelines goal for total fat and provided 24 percent of the daily, recommended intake for energy. These researchers concluded that schools on American Indian reservations are serving nutritious meals and making progress toward meeting the USDA School Meals Initiative.

Pareo-Tubbeh et al. (2000) explored the variety, affordability and availability of healthful foods at convenience stores and trading posts on the Navajo Reservation. These researchers visited 46 stores (located in New Mexico, Arizona and Utah) to record price and availability. They found that while there were improvements in the availability of healthful foods from previous studies, a limited number of such foods were available at the local trading posts that are the primary, and in most cases, the only readily accessible source of purchased food. Very few stores had low fat dairy products available; the fresh fruits and vegetables in some of the stores were in poor condition, and the prices of the healthful food varied dramatically among the stores. Some storeowners mentioned that they had carried a wider variety of perishable fruits and vegetables in the past, but had lost money due to limited demand.

Charles-Azure and Little (2005) point out that several studies have found that AI/AN adolescents consume soft drinks at more than twice the U.S. national average rate (Ballew et al., 1997). Negative consequences of this behavior include tooth decay, overweight and obesity, low bone mass, and caffeine dependence. For example, they report that oral disease rates in AI/ANs are two to three times those of the non-Indian population. Additionally, they reported on several strategies than Indian communities are implementing to reduce soft drink consumption; for example, in Fort Peck Montana, students boycotted school lunch to get soda machines replaced with bottles of water and to get a salad bar; the Hopi Nation has replaced unhealthy drinks in vending machines with healthier ones; and the Alaska Native Tribal Health Consortium and the Alaska Native Health Board started a health campaign to heighten awareness of the harmful effects of sugared soda consumption.

Charles-Azure and Little point out that it is important to plan intervention strategies that are consistent with the local traditional values; for example, a locally held focus group consisting of tribal community members could provide the direction for these types of interventions. Furthermore, they emphasize the importance of involving parents, teachers, students, families, grocers/vendors, law enforcement, health professionals, and others involved in community programs in discussions about the promotion of healthier food and beverage choices.

Food Assistance Programs

Four food assistance programs operated by USDA and one administered by DHHS (AoA) specifically designate low income AI/AN households living on or near Indian reservations as beneficiaries (Finegold et al., 2005):

- *Special Supplemental Food Program for Women, Infants and Children* (WIC). This program provides food supplements and nutrition education to low-income pregnant, breastfeeding, post-partum, and nonbreastfeeding women; infants; and children. Federal regulations allow tribes to administer WIC. In FY 2003, tribes or Indian Tribal Organizations (ITOs) administered 34 WIC programs with a combined enrollment of 60,818 (USDA, 2006). Cole (2002) estimated that 65 percent of AI pregnant women, and 48 percent of AI infants and children were enrolled in WIC. These estimates suggest that participation rates among those eligible are high.

- *Food Distribution Program on American Indian Reservations (FDPIR).* The FDPIR administered by USDA's Food and Nutrition Service (FNS) provides monthly food packages, and is an alternative to the Food Stamp Program (FSP) when access to FSP offices or authorized food stores may be a problem. Two hundred forty six tribes receive benefits under this program through 97 ITOs and 5 state agencies, but the program is not available in Alaska. FNS provides nutrition information, and the administering agencies are responsible for providing nutrition education to the participants. FNS provides the funds for these and other program administrative costs (USDA, 2005). Participants can tailor their food package by making selections within a food group and electing not to receive the fats and sweeteners. It is estimated that the current package meets or exceeds the RDA for food energy and many key nutrients. However, the package also provides several high-fat foods (U.S. GAO, 1989). Despite recent improvements, average monthly participation in 2005 dropped to 99,000, a 32 percent decline from the FY 1987 peak of 146,000, and 24 percent below the 130,000 average for FY 1999 (USDA 2004c). Additional information about current implementation of this program can be found in the USDA section of this report.
- *Food Stamp Program (FSP).* This program provides low income households with coupons or electronic benefits they can use like cash at most grocery stores. FSP is operated by state and local welfare agencies (not tribes), and the federal government oversees state operations and sets income and resource standards. Eligible households may participate in either FSP or FDPIR, but not both. In FY 2002, a monthly average of 303,000 AIs participated (Rosso & Faux, 2003). Of the various food assistance programs offered to AIs, the FDPIR and FSP are the most widely used.
- *Commodity Supplemental Food Program (CSFP).* The Commodity Supplemental Food Program (CSFP) provides packages of USDA commodity foods (rather than vouchers) to the same target group as WIC and senior citizens (60 + years of age). Recipients must meet income requirements and reside in a participating state or a reservation. More than 87 percent of current CSFP participants are elderly (USDA 2004b). The program is currently authorized to

operate in 32 states and DC; two ITOs substitute for their states in administering this program on their reservations.

- Nutrition Services Incentive Program (NSIP). Title VI of the OAA authorizes ITO participation in this program that serves the elderly and includes both congregate and home-delivered meals. Unlike other USDA programs, Native Hawaiian organizations can quality for ITO status and administer the NSIP.

Programs that do not specifically identify AIs as participants, but serve Indians on reservations include: National School Lunch and Breakfast Programs, Child and Adult Care Food Program, Special Milk Program, and Summer Food Service Program.

Studies of reservation food assistance programs have found large numbers of participants for whom these programs are the main, or even the only, source of food. Miller (1994), for example, in studying all seven reservations in Montana (N=1,356), reported that the FDPIR was the main source of food for 51.5 percent of households participating in this program, and the only source of food for 7.4 percent. More recently, Hiwalker et al. (2002) found that the major sources of food on the Northern Cheyenne Reservation (Montana) were wages (64 percent of respondents), the FDPIR (33 percent), Food Stamps (31 percent) and WIC (26 percent). All those interviewed said that when they could, they shared with neighbors, family, and friends in need of food.

Dillinger et al. (1999) studied 80 families and their use of supplemental food programs in a rural and an urban tribal community in California. Fifty-eight percent of rural respondents, but only 20 percent of the urban respondents used food commodities. This is explainable in part because distribution of food commodities in rural areas is direct to clients, while in urban areas, clients must travel to food banks and closets to obtain these commodities. Furthermore, in urban areas, 51 percent the Native American respondents were unfamiliar with the food programs compared to 2 percent in the rural community. While urban residents had access to more sources of food assistance and nutrition education than rural residents, access to nutrition counseling was inadequate at both sites. Healthier foods (e.g., fresh fruits and vegetables and meats) were either lacking or in short supply. The authors stated that these programs may create unhealthy food preferences among rural and urban Native Americans. They recommended complementary nutrition programs, fresh produce, nutrition counseling, accommodation of Native American food preferences, and use of potlucks and seasonal assemblies for nutrition education.

In their background report on food assistance programs on Indian reservations, Finegold et al. (2005) point to several key issues regarding these programs:

- *Quality of FDPIR and Relationship to Obesity*. FDPIR food packages were updated in FY 1998 and distribution continues to improve making the program healthier and more consumer-friendly than it was. Thus, the effects of the program on health and nutritional outcomes may be better than in the past (Fox et al., 2004). Tribal administrators of the commodity programs have noticed improvements in the content, quality, and variety of foods offered, but say that the ingredients of the products could still be made healthier. Apart from the factors affecting choice between FDPIR and FSP, we do not really know whether one or the other of these programs produces better health and nutritional outcomes.
  Currently participants may select from over 70 products each month, and tribes may opt to receive fresh produce distributed to households in lieu of canned fruits and vegetables. Seventy-two percent of the tribes participating have elected and been approved to participate in the fresh produce program (IHS, 2001). Many tribes have better facilities for food storage than in the past, allowing them to offer more fresh foods.
  Reservation residents developed the term "commod bod" to describe the physique of AIs who relied heavily on commodity packages that were high in fat and highly sweetened (Welty 1991; Dillinger et al., 1999). Many low-income individuals are both overweight and participants in one or more nutrition assistance programs. This has led some to question whether participation in the nutrition assistance programs contributes to the growing problem of overweight and obesity. In order to determine the relationship between obesity and program participation, it is necessary to separate the effects of poverty and socioeconomic class from the effects of food assistance, but because poverty is highly correlated with program participation, it is difficult to separate their independent effects (Finegold et al., 2005).
  A review of existing research (USDA, 2004a) found no evidence that there is an empirical basis for a causal relationship among any of the four major nutrition assistance programs -- FSP, WIC, National School Lunch Program (NSLP), and the School Breakfast Program

(SBP) – and obesity, and no evidence that program participation causes obesity. For example, there is no published research that considers the relationship between participation in the WIC program and maternal obesity or participation in the NSLP and SBP and overweight/obesity. While the published research on Food Stamps indicates there is some association between program participation and overweight/obesity, there is no evidence of causality. Existing studies are limited by not controlling for food insecurity, an important intervening variable, or relying on cross- sectional data.

- *Traditional Foods and Practices.* Many tribal leaders have expressed their desire that the commodity packages provide more traditional foods. This would demonstrate, they say, that USDA is responsive to tribal desires and would also have a positive economic impact for the localities. In response, FDPIR has offered bison meat to program participants since FY 2001. However, the FDPIR Food Package Work Group determined that some culturally preferred foods (e.g., blue cornmeal) were much more expensive and provided no nutritional advantage over the product current offered (i.e., yellow cornmeal).

  Studies of the Ojibwa and Tohono O'odham tribes reported limited availability of traditional foods that would support a healthy diet. Several nutritional initiatives have been designed to improve access to such foods. For example, the Ojibwa project planned to produce a cookbook of traditional foods and encourage local restaurants and feeding programs to incorporate traditional foods in their menus (Parrish, 2002). The Apache Healthy Stores project, funded by USDA, works with grocery stores on Arizona's White Mountain and San Carlos Reservations to promote healthy foods.

  An issue applicable to all of the food assistance programs is how the programs interact with tribal norms, such as the sharing of food. Alives (1993) observed that multigenerational, extended families were valuable networks for her Extension Service work with the Navajo Nation. Similarly, Smith and Wiedman (2000), found that program endorsement by female elders was the key to connecting eligible mothers with WIC services in an Aleutian community. Dillinger et al. (1999) identified potlucks and powwows as good opportunities for nutrition education.

- *Nutrition Education and Counseling.* For all of the food assistance programs, diet-related health problems raise questions about how much to spend on nutrition education and how to design effective, culturally appropriate nutrition education programs in which AIs will be able and willing to participate. Shanklin et al. (1992) found that in 1980, 8 of 30 FDPIR programs surveyed reported no spending on nutritional education, and only 2 of the 30 programs had full-time nutrition coordinators on staff. The recent Finegold et al. (2005) study found that tribal administrators repeatedly cite program literature received from the USDA as their main source of nutritional information.

- *Coordination among Programs.* An issue affecting all the food assistance programs is how they can be better integrated with each other and with non-USDA programs such as Temporary Assistance for Needy Families (TANF), IHS, and the economic development programs of the Bureau of Indian Affairs. Increased coordination could improve participation, access, availability, and effectiveness of nutrition education. Some have raised questions about the level of coordination between the FDPIR and the FSP. Because one program is administered by tribes and the other is not, it is not possible for one worker on the reservation to counsel clients and facilitate enrollment for both programs. The transportation problems of many Indians living on reservations make the idea of a single, tribally administered site for all low-income programs appealing (Finegold et al., 2005).

Socioeconomic Factors

Kumanyika and Grier (2006) point out that making progress in the fight against childhood obesity in racial and ethnic minority and low income communities will depend on our national will to radically alter the negative effects of the social and physical environments in which these communities exist. They review evidence that indicate the higher rates of obesity in these communities are associated with a plethora of unfavorable influences – economic stresses, reduced access to affordable healthful foods, opportunities for safe and varied physical activity, overexposure to targeted advertising, and marketing of energy-dense foods. Thus, they indicate that simply counseling parents and children about weight control will be almost pointless in environments with these characteristics.

The Surgeon General's Call to Action to Prevent and Decrease Overweight and Obesity (DHHS, 2001) states that disparities in the prevalence of overweight and obesity exist based on socioeconomic status. For all racial and ethnic groups combined, women of lower socioeconomic status (SES) are approximately 50 percent more likely to be obese than those with higher SES. Men are about equally likely to be obese whether they are in a low or high SES group.

Unemployment and poverty have continuously plagued the vast majority of Native American communities. In 1999, the poverty rate for AI/ANs was 25.7 percent compared to 12.4 percent for the total population. AI/ANs participate in the labor force at a lower rate than the total population, and labor force participation varies by tribal groupings. In 2000, this participation for AI/AN men was 66 percent compared to 71 percent for all men, while labor force participation for AI/AN women was 57 percent compared to 58 percent for all women. Also, in 2000, the median earnings of AI/AN men ($28,900) and women ($22,800) who worked full time, year-round were substantially below those of all men ($37,100) and women ($27,200) (U.S. Census Bureau, 2006).

Furthermore, the educational levels of AI/ANs were below those of the total population in 2000; 71 percent of AI/ANs 25 years and older had at least a high school education, compared with 80 percent of the total population. Eleven percent of AI/ANs had at least a bachelor's degree compared with 24 percent of all people (U.S. Census Bureau, 2006).

These socioeconomic circumstances of AI/AN/s affect their general living conditions, ability to find employment, types of foods they are able to purchase, resources available for exercise and recreational activities, and overall physical and emotional health. While the circumstances of each tribe are unique, most tribes have experienced economic, education, housing, health, and other problems at levels of severity rarely seen in most other American communities. These problems are long-standing, and they reflect unique historical and cultural factors as well as socioeconomic ones (Hillabrant et al., 2001).

Psychosocial Factors

Historical Trauma

Historical trauma and grief are sometimes cited as factors impacting psychological and physical health and contributing to the health disparities between AI/ANs and other groups. Brave Heart indicates that historical trauma has a layering effect and defines the concept as the collective emotional and psychological injury both over the life span and across generations resulting from the history of difficulties that Native Americans as a group have experienced in America (Steinman, 2005). These experiences are not "historical" in the sense that they are in the past and a new life has begun in a new land. Rather, the losses are ever present, represented by the economic conditions of reservation life, discrimination, and a sense of cultural loss (Whitbeck et al., 2004).

The symptoms of historical trauma identified by Brave Heart and colleagues run the gamut of those associated with post-traumatic stress disorder to symptoms of unresolved grief. However, many of the symptoms overlap and their number encompasses almost the entire range of psychopathology. Feelings associated with these losses include anger, a deep and persistent depression, intrusiveness of these thoughts, discomfort around White people, and fearl and distrust of the intentions of White people (Brave Heart, 1998 & 1998a). Whitebeck et al., found that historical trauma and historical grief were prevalent among the contemporary parent generation and not confined to the more proximate elder generation (Whitbeck et al., 2004).

There has been very little research done in this area. In the first systematic assessment of the prevalence of trauma exposure in AI communities, Manson et al. (2005) found that unlike the U.S. general population, female and male AIs from one southwest and two northern plains tribes exhibited equivalent levels of overall trauma exposure (females had less in the general population studies). Members of these tribes more often witnessed traumatic events, experienced traumas to loved ones, and were victims of physical attacks compared to their counterparts in the overall U.S. population. They concluded that AIs live in adverse environments that place them at high risk for exposure to trauma and harmful health sequelae.

Perception of Obesity

Adults. Weight attitudes, norms, body image concepts, and standards of attractiveness are believed to be strongly influenced by sociocultural factors; however, it is unclear whether AI/AN communities view obesity as a health problem (Story et al., 2003; Broussard et al., 1995; Ghodes, 1995). In her discussion of obesity in minority populations, Kumanyika (1995) notes that persons in racial/ethnic populations appear to be more likely to place some positive or neutral value on obesity compared to persons in White populations whose attitudes may be more uniformly negative. The effect of these more mixed cultural values, she says, may offer some protection from the extreme fear or stigmatization of obesity that can contribute to eating disorders in the larger culture. A dynamic that may operate in AI/AN communities is that a tipping point with regard to community normalization of obesity and/or resignation may be reached when 50 percent or more of the population are overweight/obese (Cullen, 2006).

White et al. (1997) in their study of the Navajos found that men and women age 60 and older chose overweight images as ideals of health more often than younger participants. They concluded that older Navajo clients believe that moderate overweight is normal and healthy. Similarly, Teufel and Dufour (1990) studying a small sample of 28 Hualapai Indian women in northwest Arizona found that obesity did not have negative social consequences. The women reported eating alone and eating large quantities of food. These researchers suggested that AI women may be more candid than middle-class Anglo-Americans when evaluating serving size, frequency of consumptions, food preference and selection, and methods of preparation.

The topic of obesity/overweight may be a sensitive issue for medical professionals serving AI/ANs. In the past, doctors themselves may not have known what to do about this issue, but, they have more to say about obesity today, and it is important that they say it so they believe it (Cullen, 2006). Reid and Rhoades (2000) note that a seldom-discussed component of present- day Indian life is the element of shame. Any sign of approbation or judgment on the part of the health-care provider is apt to stimulate this feeling, to the detriment of the interview. They note that Indians are extremely sensitive about references to them having high rates of poverty, alcoholism, and other diseases.

Youth. In studying a large sample of 11,868 youth in 7th-12th grades residing in eight Indian Health Service (IHS) areas, Neumark-Sztainer et al. (1997) concluded that the weak and inconsistent associations they found between overweight status and global psychological and social concerns (e.g., suicidal ideation, peer or future job concerns) suggest greater acceptance of overweight youth in this culture, or at least that being overweight has a limited impact on psychosocial health.

Davis et al. (1993), in their study of 1,527 5th grade AI children, referred to a commonly held belief that AI people value obesity as highly desirable and therefore are not amenable to health education efforts that focus on preventing or reducing obesity. However, these researchers found that although this belief may have been true in the past and may still be true for some adults, the children they studied were aware of their body size and cognizant of the importance of maintaining a moderate weight. They found that although 67 percent of these children's families did not own a scale, the children had an accurate perception of their weight. Fifty-nine percent of the youngsters reported they had tried to lose weight, and the majority of these youngsters were aware that increasing exercise was one way to do this.

Several of the key informants from the Gila River Indian Community indicated that obese adults are accepted among Native Americans. The community members explained it this way: "Someone who is skinny is perceived as not doing well. If someone is thin, others will say, "You need to fatten up" or ask them "Are you OK?" Other respondents from this tribe indicated that the culture prizes largeness. They stated that being big is a part of one's identity and is equated with any of the following: being healthy, a good farmer, a sign of wealth, or sexual attractiveness.

Depression

Daniels (2006) observes that discerning the direction of the relationship between obesity and depression is difficult. He says that depression itself is often associated with abnormal patterns of eating and physical activity that could result in future obesity; however, obesity may also result in psychosocial problems that can produce depression. He indicates that the evidence supports both hypotheses; for example youths with depression are at greater risk to develop an increased BMI, and higher BMI has also been linked with increasing symptoms of depression in elementary school girls (Pine et al., 2001; Eisenberg et al., 2003).

There are few studies that discuss depression in relation to obesity among AI/ANs. In one survey of 458 Northern Plains Indians that focused on the role of nutrition and physical activity in the development and course of chronic disease and depression, findings indicated that depression (measurement and definition unclear) was strongly associated with measures of generalized distress. These researchers also found that depression was associated with poorer health, less exercise, food insecurity, and tobacco use in males and females. Depression scores were higher in those reporting lower income, more children and food insecurity, while these scores were lower in those reporting stronger identity with native culture and language (Bliss, 2004).

Although studies that associated obesity with depression were not located, a few studies address the prevalence of mental disorders among AI/ANs. In an analysis of data from the 2001-2002 National Epidemiological Survey of Alcohol and Related Conditions (N=43,000), findings indicated that Native American race was one of the factors that increased the likelihood of Major Depressive Disorder (MDD). And, among race groups, Native Americans showed the highest (19.17%) lifetime MDD prevalence followed by Whites (14.58), Hispanics (9.64), Blacks (8.93) and Asian or Pacific Islanders (8.77) (Hasin et al., 2006). We know that AI/ANs die at a rate 62 percent higher than other Americans from suicide (IHS, 2006), but the research literature does not directly connect obesity with this problem. In another study of a Northern Plains tribe and a Southwest tribe (N=3,000), Arehart-Treichel (2005) found that these tribes were at greater lifetime risk for posttraumatic stress disorder and alcohol dependence than the general American population. However, unlike the Hasin et al., study, this study found that both of the Indian tribes had a lower lifetime risk of major depression than the general American population

Genetic Factors

Historically, for Pima Indians and many other cultures, periods of abundant food have alternated with periods of famine. A "thrifty gene" might have enabled individuals to store surplus calories as fat during times of abundance and to use the energy more efficiently during times of famine, thus surviving periods when food was scarce. This gene was helpful as long as there were periods of famine, but once these populations adopted the typical Western lifestyle, with less physical activity, a high fat diet, and access to a constant supply of calories, this gene began to work against them, continuing to store calories in preparation for famine but contributing to unhealthy amounts of fat. It was Neel (1962) who developed a hypothesis to explain this pattern, suggesting that obesity is the expression of a "thrifty gene" that conferred an evolutionary advantage in a subsistence lifestyle, but which became detrimental with progress.

The role of genetics in relation to the environment is complex and is an area where there is disagreement. Ravussin (1995) explains that environment explains weight differences when populations with similar genetic backgrounds are living in different environments (e.g., Pima Tribes in the U.S. are heavier than those Pimas living in Mexico), while genetics can help explain differences in weight within populations living in a similar environment (e.g., Pimas living in the Southwest U.S). Studies (of individuals of all races) on twins reared apart, siblings and adopted twins within a given environment have found a genetic factor associated with obesity in individuals of all races. For further information on research pertaining to the Pima Indians, refer to the Gila River Indian Community section of this paper under National Institute of Diabetes, Digestive and Kidney Diseases (NIDDK) Research Presentations.

Research evidence appears mixed regarding genetic factors in relation to obesity in AIs. In her review, Story et al. (2003) noted that there was little evidence to support a role of energy expenditure in the development of childhood obesity, as neither energy expenditure nor metabolic rate is significantly different between AI and White children (Fontvieille et al., 1993; Goran et al., 1995). However, other researchers identified three metabolic predictors of obesity in Pima Indians, a group that has a high prevalence of obesity and diabetes: low metabolic rates (Walston et al., 1995; Ravussin, 1995), a high 24-hour respiratory quotient (Zurlo et al., 1990, Ravussin, 1995), and insulin sensitivity (Swinburn et al., 1991, Ravussin, 1995). Additionally, North et al. (2003) found in studying 950 American Indians in Arizona, Oklahoma and the Dakotas (Strong Heart Family Study) that there may be different genes operating in diabetic and nondiabetic patients for several obesity [e.g., body mass index, body fat mass] and lipid-related risk factors, but indicate that future research is needed to more closely examine these findings.

Weiss et al. (1992) put the thrifty gene hypothesis in a broader context when they described the "New World Syndrome," a complex of conditions with high prevalence among AIs. These conditions include obesity, gallstones, gallbladder cancer, abnormalities of cholesterol metabolism, and non-insulin type 2 diabetes. They hypothesized that these co-occurring conditions increase together in prevalence in AIs in proportion to the degree of modernization of life-style and suggested that some underlying abnormality in lipid metabolism must be responsible for the syndrome, in interaction with modern diet and exercise patterns. While the research noted above has examined whether genetic factors play a role in the etiology of obesity, Ravussin (1995), Story et al. (2003), and Harrison & Ritenbaugh (1992) point out that genetic and environmental factors may interact; for example, the environment plays a role either by compounding a genetic tendency toward weight gain or by mitigating it.

Physical Activity

Adults

Physical activity is protective against obesity and other health risks, but in the process of acculturation, AI/ANs have shifted from a traditional subsistence lifestyle to a more sedentary one that involves much less physical activity (Mendlein et al., 1997; Sugarman, 1992).

Using the National Health Information Survey to compare AI/ANs to other ethnic groups, Barnes et al. (2005) they found that AI/AN adults (50.3 percent) were as likely as Black adults (49.9 percent) and more likely than Asian adults (38.1 percent) and White adults (36.6 percent) to never engage in any leisure-time physical activity. Also, AI/AN adults (26.2 percent) were as likely as Asian adults (29.0) and Black adults (24.4 percent), but less likely than White adults (33.1 percent) to engage in regular leisure time physical activity.

There have been only limited studies of physical activity among AI/ANs. The Navajo Health and Nutrition survey (Mendlein et al., 1997) and the Strong Heart Study (Yurgalevitch et al., 1998) that targeted adults age 45-74 found low physical activity levels among those living on reservation-based communities. Specific barriers to physical activity that were cited by respondents include limited child care; lack of time; and safety concerns such as fear of traffic, snakes and dogs when walking; and lack of willpower or motivation (Harnack et al., 1999). Additionally, Phillips and Finn (2000) found that among the Lakota Sioux (Cheyenne River Sioux Reservation in South Dakota), the primary barrier to regular exercise was poor accessibility to the Tribal Fitness Center that has limited facilities especially during after work hours. Also, several respondents in this study indicated that an individual's medical conditions or disabilities were barriers, and that these conditions required exercise equipment or non-impact exercise such as swimming.

The majority of respondents in a study of Hopi (Giuliano et al., 1998) and Lakota adults (Harnack et al., 1999) indicated that they engaged in mild or moderate physical activities to keep healthy; however, several of these studies found that that men were more physically active than women (Yurgalevitch et al., 1998; Harnack et al., 1999) or that healthy behaviors including exercise were practiced more frequently as women (ages18-89) became older (Giuliano et al., 1998). These findings resulted in recommendations to target health promotion/education efforts to women or younger women. Additionally, the findings suggested environmental interventions are needed to increase opportunities for physical activity and address barriers on reservations; for example, family-oriented physical activities, child care allowing adults to leave their children to exercise, community centers, outdoor walking trails, and school gymnasiums open for community use (Harnack et al., 1999).

One study conducted by Powell et al. (2004) focused specifically on the environment as it is related to physical activity using a nationally representative sample of 409 communities. These researchers made use of outdoor observational data pertaining to community-level physical activity-related settings (such as sports areas or parks) as well as Census Bureau data. They found that the availability of environmental factors that are conducive to physical activity such as sports areas, parks and green spaces, public pools and beaches, and the presence of bike paths/lanes are significantly associated with racial, ethnic and socioeconomic status (SES) factors. Overall, these results suggest that communities with low SES populations and higher proportions of minority racial groups who are most at risk of inactivity and overweight are also associated with the fewest community-level physical activity-related settings. Hence targeted interventions to improve access to neighborhood physical activity-related opportunities may help to reduce the persistent disparities in health related to SES. Interventions should include proactive urban planning policies to reduce barriers related to physical activity (Powell et al., 2004).

Two interesting studies compare activity patterns between Mexican Indians and U.S. Indians – groups that may be genetically similar but live in different environments and have dissimilar lifestyles. Esparza et al. (2000) measured total energy expenditure in age and sex matched cohorts of 40 Mexican and 40 U.S Pima Indians. The Mexican Pimas were lighter, leaner and nondiabetic compared to the U.S Pimas. In fact, the Pima Indians of Arizona have been found to be particularly prone to obesity (Knowler et al., 1991). Findings indicated that physical activity was greater among the Mexican Pimas. They continue to live a traditional lifestyle in the Sierra Madre Mountains, while the U.S. Pimas live a typical North American lifestyle. The Mexican Pimas spent more time on occupational activities that were physical (e.g., wood milling, non- mechanized farming), while farming for the U.S. Pimas is mechanized and their physical activities are less frequent and of a lower intensity than their Mexican counterparts. The difference in physical activity amounted to 500-600 kcal/day. The researchers concluded that the greater energy expenditure in combination with a diet lower in fat and higher in fiber may protect the Mexican Pimas against obesity and type 2 diabetes.

Similarly, Conner et al. (1978) also found that the unwesternized Tarahumara tribe of Mexico when compared to the Yaquis Indians of Arizona (migrated from Mexico in the early 20th century) had low levels of obesity and cardiovascular disease risks, but also higher levels of physical activity along with diets that were lower in fat.

In a study examining physical activity and lipids in older reservation-based AI adults 45-74 years of age (N=4,249) in Arizona (AZ), Oklahoma (OK), and South and North Dakota (S/ND), researchers found differences between those living in the various geographic areas of the U.S. (Yurgalevitch et al., 1998). They found the least amount of leisure and occupational physical activity (during the past year) reported by the men and women living in Arizona, and this group also had the highest percentage of participants reporting no leisure activity, a finding in agreement with previous investigations of the activity levels of Pima Indians. For example, 53 percent, 32 percent, and 32 percent of men from AZ, OK and S/ND respectively reported participating in no leisure physical activity over the past week, and 60 percent, 42 percent and 40 percent of the women from these same areas reported the same finding. In comparison with activity levels of the general U.S. population of similar ages, the AIs living in the Arizona communities had substantially lower levels of physical activity.

Youth

Gray and Smith (2003) studied *urban* Anishinaabe-Ojibwe youth in Minnesota ages 5-18 (N=155). They found that 59 percent of these youth were sedentary. Body mass index was correlated with physical activity and frequency of TV viewing. TV viewing averaged 3.9 hours per day, with 13-18 year olds watching the greatest amount of TV. These authors recommend that culturally appropriate interventions for obesity should start early focusing on reducing sedentary activity and increasing opportunities for fitness. In another study, Fontvieille et al. (1993) reported that Pima Indian boys and girls (average age of 10) spent significantly less time engaged in sport leisure activities and more time watching television than their non-Indian counterparts. Since the Pima children had higher levels of obesity than the Caucasian children, the researchers associated obesity with decreased physical activity and increased television watching, although the nature of the causal relationship is not clear.

In a formative assessment of six tribes and nine schools during the feasibility phase of the Pathways Study (a school-based obesity prevention intervention with AI/ANs), Thompson et al. (2001) used surveys, interviews and direct observation to examine barriers to physical activity within the elementary school environment itself. They found a lack of facilities, equipment and trained physical education staff. Furthermore, very few schools reported before or after class activities held at the school. Additionally, most family members or child caregivers said they did not participate in exercise or physical activities; however, parents were supportive of their children's activities by driving them to these activities. The barriers that these adults cited as contributing to their lack of physical activity included: embarrassment, lack of exercise facilities and financial resources, working long hours, and a history of illnesses such as diabetes. The authors of this study recommended that parents do the following: work with schools and teachers to insist that physical activity opportunities are available at school, provide physical activity opportunities for children outside of school, and be physically active with their children.

Consequences of Obesity

Physical Health Consequences

Although the AI/ANs are not a homogeneous group with regard to physical health problems, they have all suffered adverse effects from the high prevalence of obesity (Welty, 1991). These health risks are well documented; thus, this paper will focus only briefly on this topic, targeting diabetes and cardiovascular disease (CVD) key consequences for adults and youth.

Adults

Known obesity-related health risks for adults include increased likelihood of type 2 diabetes, hypertension, cardiovascular disease, and problems with lipid levels (NRCCDH, 1989). These risks are higher for people with centralized body fat (e.g. abdominal fat) than for people with peripheral body fat (Howard et al., 1995). Obesity also increases the risk of mortality for adults of all races from gallbladder cancer, endometrial cancer in women and colorectal cancer in men (NRCCDH, 1989).

The association of type 2 diabetes with obesity in AI/AN populations is well known (Lee et al., 1995, Welty, 1991). For example, in the Strong Heart Study of AI/AN adults, the rate of diabetes increased steadily with BMI in both sexes (Lee et al., 1995). During 1996-1998, the AI/AN age-adjusted death rates for diabetes were 3.9 times the rate for U.S. all races (U.S. DHHS, 2005).

Furthermore, diabetes rates have increased over time. A study by the Centers for Disease Control and Prevention of the IHS national outpatient database found nearly a 30 percent increase in diabetes diagnoses among AI/AN populations between 1990-1997. The increase in prevalence was highest in Alaska where it rose by 76 percent and lowest in the Northern Plains region where it rose by 16 percent (Burrows et al., 2000). It is estimated that half of all type 2 diabetes is preventable by obesity control (McGinnis & Foege, 1993).

Obesity is an independent risk factor for CVD heart disease. In the Strong Heart Study of AI/ANs, the prevalence of CVD in AIs was significantly and independently related to percentage of body fat as well as other factors (Howard et al., 1995). Obesity is also a risk factor for hypertension, and hypertension in turn is a risk factor for CVD, coronary artery disease, stroke and peripheral vascular disease. IHS reports in the latest *Trends in Indian Health* report covering 1996-1998 (U.S. DHHS, 2005), that diseases of the heart are the leading cause of death for AI/ANs in several age groups including 45-54, 55-64, and 65+ as well as for AI/ANs of all ages. However, CVD mortality rates and the prevalence of CVD risk factors vary between AI tribes (Story et al., 1999).

Youth

Obesity is a hallmark of type 2 diabetes with up to 85 percent of children either overweight or obese at diagnosis (Story et al., 2003). There has been a recent significant increase in the prevalence of type 2 diabetes among AI youth in the U.S; this condition is now commonly seen in AI children aged 10 and over (Dabelea et al., 1998; Fagot-Campagna et al., 2000). An IHS study found that from 1990-1998, the prevalence of diabetes increased by 68 percent among adolescents 15-19 years; however, the prevalence among children younger than 15 years remained unchanged (Acton et al., 2002). Children who develop type 2 diabetes are at greater risk for various health complications compared to those diagnosed as adults (Story et al., 2003).

Childhood overweight increases the risk of adult overweight, the clustering of other CVD risk factors, coronary calcification in adulthood, and all cause CVD mortality (Power et al., 1997). Several researchers have reported a relationship between obesity and high blood pressure in AI youth (Gilbert et al., 1992; Smith & Rinderknecht, 2003). For example, Smith & Rinderknecht found in studying 155 urban AI youth ages 5-18 years that increased BMI is correlated with elevated systolic and diastolic blood pressures that may put these youth at risk of CVD in the future. Furthermore, both Blackett et al. (1996) and Freedman et al. (1997) found in studying 103 Oklahoma Indian children ages 4-19 years and in Navajo adolescents 12-19 years respectively that BMI was associated with elevated lipid levels (e.g., higher cholesterol and higher triglyceride levels).

Psychosocial Consequences

Overweight and obese individuals may suffer from social stigmatization, discrimination, poor body image, and in some studies poor self-esteem (U.S.

DHHS, 2001; Dietz, 1998; Must & Strauss, 1999), and obese children and adolescents have difficulties with peer relationships (Strauss & Pollack, 2006). It is believed that these psychosocial consequences result from the societal value placed on thinness as the ideal body form. However, the majority of studies in this area have been done with White populations; thus it is unclear whether or to what extent there may be adverse psychological effects related to obesity in AI adults or youth (Story et al., 2003). The studies discussed below pertain specifically to AI/ANs and discuss knowledge and locus of control, concern with obesity/overweight, and weight-loss practices.

Adults

Knowledge and Locus of Control. Harnack et al. (1995) and Sherwood et al. (2000) in studying 219 Lakota adult Indians residing on a South Dakota reservation and 203 urban adult Indian women residing in the Minneapolis/St. Paul area found that respondents understood that obesity, diabetes, heart disease, and hypertension/high blood pressure are related to dietary behavior. They also found that respondents believe that people have control over their weight, i.e., have an internal locus of control. Similarly Hood et al. (1997) found in assessing the Mohawk Community of Akwesasne in New York that the major identifiable barriers were not a lack of knowledge of healthy dietary practices and the value of exercise, but preferences for high fat foods and their ready availability, desire for large servings, and less physically active lifestyles. And, perhaps more important, they found that a lack of confidence for personal lifestyle change, a lack of skills needed to bring about this change, and a lack of social support for these efforts were critical barriers.

Concern about Weight and Weight-Loss Practices. Several researchers found that AIs are concerned about their weight and are engaging in practices to lose weight (Harnack et al., 1999; Sherwood et al., 2000). For example, Harnack et al., found that those who were overweight were more likely to diet one or more times in the past year (58 percent of those overweight versus 38 percent of the non-overweight). Furthermore, White et al. (1997) found in studying 788 Navaho adults, that among both men and women, trying to lose weight was most common among those 20-39 years, less common among those 40-59 years and least common among those 60+. Additionally, among those 20-39 years and those age 60+, women reported trying to lose weight more often than men. Harnack et al., concluded that because this population was aware of and concerned about obesity/overweight as a problem, strategies need not dwell on convincing this population that the problem of obesity exists. Rather, the focus should be on effective strategies for weight loss or obesity prevention.

Several studies have found that of those who felt they needed a weight-loss program, the majority said they would like to join one if it were offered in their community (Harnack et al., 1999; Sherwood et al., 2000; Phillips and Finn, 2000). However, the majority of Sherwood and colleagues sample (90.1 percent) had never participated in an organized weight-loss program. These authors found that the following factors were important to respondents in considering joining a weight-loss program; offered at no cost, provision of food, friends to join with, transportation, available child care, and programs offered at worksites.

Unhealthful Practices. While healthy weight loss practices were practiced most frequently, both Harnack et al., and Sherwood et al., found that some AIs in their urban and reservation-based samples reported undesirable dieting practices. For example, Sherwood et al., found that 33 percent of their sample (N=203) fasted, 15 percent used diet pills or smoking more cigarettes as strategies, 6 percent used self-induced vomiting, and 33 percent reported binge eating. They concluded that 9 percent of their entire sample may have had clinically notable binge eating problems, and the majority of these self-reported binge eaters were overweight. These researchers report that this rate is higher than those typically observed in community samples, but comparable to what is observed among those in weight loss programs in the general population.

Youth

Knowledge. Rinderknecht and Smith (2002) found in studying 155 urban AI children 5-18 years of age that these youth identified the heavy body shapes that were most likely to develop diabetes; thus, they appeared to understand that obesity may create long-term health problems.

Concern about Weight and Weight Loss Practices. Studies with AI youths, particularly girls show that they are dissatisfied with their weight, worry about being overweight, attempt to lose weight, and use unhealthy weight control methods (Story et al., 2003; Davis and Lambert, 2000; Story et al., 2001; Neumark-Sztainter et al., 1997).

For example, the Indian Adolescent Health survey, including more than 13,454 7th-12th grade nonurban youth from eight IHS service areas, found that 50 percent of the adolescent girls were dissatisfied with their weight, and 44 percent were worried about being overweight. Almost half the girls had been on a weight-loss diet in the past year. When these researchers compared the AI youth to rural White youths from Minnesota, both the AI girls and boys had greater dissatisfaction with their body weight than the Minnesota youth. (Story et al., 1994). Story et al. (2001) found in their sample of 1441 second and third grade AI children representing 7 tribes that heavier children (especially those with BMI > 95) were more likely to have tried to lose weight or were currently trying to lose weight.

Similarly, Neumark-Sztainer et al. (1997) found that the older overweight AI youth who were concerned about their weight were somewhat less likely than nonoverweight youth to engage in health-promoting behaviors such as fruit and vegetable consumption and regular exercise. Overall, in their AI sample (N=11,868) these researchers found weak and inconsistent associations between overweight status and psychosocial concerns (i.e., suicidal ideation, future job concerns, and peer concerns) suggesting that "greater social acceptance of overweight in this culture, or at least that overweight has a limited impact on psychosocial health." They concluded that since the prevalence of psychosocial concerns and health-compromising behaviors and poor eating behaviors was high among both nonoverweight and overweight youth, obesity in their 7th-12th grade sample may best be addressed within a comprehensive health promotion framework.

Unhealthful practices. Similar to the findings pertaining to adults, Story et al. (2001) and Neumark-Sztainter et al. (1997) found unhealthy practices primarily among overweight AI youth. For example, Story et al. (2001) reported that approximately 40 percent of the overweight youth and 50 percent of the obese youth said they had gone for a day without eating to lose weight. And, results from the Indian Adolescent Health Survey indicated 27 percent of the girls reported they had self-induced vomiting at some time in an attempt to lose weight (Story et al., 1994). The Minnesota Adolescent Health Survey found that the prevalence of chronic dieting, self-induced vomiting, laxative use, binge dieting, and body pride were similar among AI girls and White girls (Story et al., 1995).

Story et al. (2001) stated that the evidence of unhealthy practices highlights the need for health education and guidance on healthy weight management practices. Furthermore, they cautioned that efforts to increase public awareness of the health risks of obesity do not increase undue concern and preoccupation, body dissatisfaction and unhealthy dieting in children and adolescents.

Salbe et al. (2002) in their longitudinal study of 138 Pima Indian children concluded that the perception that a child is overweight is apparently not sufficient to overcome other factors. They found that 67 percent of parents correctly perceived that their child was overweight at age 5 and were informed of the risks and given referrals for follow-up care. However, in only one child, did this information result in decreased risk at age 10. By the age of 5 years, almost 28 percent of these children were overweight; at the age of 10 years, 53 percent of these same children were overweight.

Economic Consequences

Further research is needed to determine economic costs associated with obesity/overweight that are specific to AI/ANs. However, we know that these conditions in the general population are associated with extensive direct (e.g., preventive, diagnostic and treatment services) and indirect costs (e.g., value of lost wages) (U.S. DHHS, 2001; U.S. News & World Report, 2005).

Intervention Research

This section will focus on a selection of published intervention research studies regarding AI/ANs and obesity prevention. Only completed studies are described; additional studies in progress are included in the IHS, NIH, CDC, and USDA sections of this report. The section begins with Table 4 that summarizes the interventions and is followed by a description of each intervention and an overall summary of the interventions.

Satterfield et al. (2003) conceptualize intervention approaches as clinical and community-based. Clinical interventions follow the “high-risk” approach which often occurs in a resource intensive clinical setting and focuses exclusively on individuals at highest risk for developing diseases. Community-based approaches follow a “population or public health” approach which attempts to reduce risk factors for or causes of diseases within communities. In addition to promoting lifestyle adaptations, these approaches can identify and support protective factors within the culture, help garner social support among family and community members, and have far-reaching influences that, along with environmental changes, can help support adaptive responses among people at various points along a continuum of risk.

Community-based interventions may be based on an ecological model that focuses on change in interpersonal processes (e.g., characteristics of the individual), interpersonal processes and primary groups (e.g., families), institutional factors (e.g., schools), community factors (e.g., social norms), and public policy (e.g., local regulations and policies).

Table 4. Interventions Related to Obesity Prevention Involving AI/ANs

Clinical Interventions						
Name of Study & Reference	**Geographic Location Target Audience Sample Size**	**Study design & duration**	**Goals**	**Intervention**	**Community Involvement/ Cultural Relevance**	**Results**
Diabetes Prevention Program (DPP) DPP Research Group, 1999)	AIs from Southwest U.S. tribes including Salt River, Zuni, Gila River Indian Community, & Navaho Tribes as well as other groups. Adults at risk of diabetes N= 3,235 (total) including 171 AIs	Randomized clinical trial 1996-2001	Determine if lifestyle intervention or drug therapy prevents or delays onset of diabetes.	Three groups: 1) Intensive lifestyle modification 2) Standard lifestyle recommendations & metformin (drug) 3) Standard lifestyle recommendations & placebo.	Lifestyle coaches from same ethnic groups as participant. Intervention strategies addressed needs of ethnically diverse populations.	No difference in treatment effects by race/ethnic group or sex. Incidence of diabetes reduced by 58% in intensive lifestyle group & by 31% in metformin group compared with placebo group. Intensive lifestyle group achieved significantly greater weight loss.
Lifestyle Interventions in Pima Indians Narayan et al., 1998	Gila River Indian Community. Arizona Pima adults who are overweight but normoglycemic. N=95 (total)	Pilot trial randomized into intervention group (IG) and comparison group (CG) 1 year	Test adherence to specific lifestyle interventions & compare them for changes in diabetes risk factors (e.g., obesity).	IG: structured physical activity & nutrition interventions; behavioral techniques e.g., group problem solving & food preparation demos CG: unstructured activities focused on history & culture. Also written info on healthy eating & exercise.	Pima community created intervention including local speakers, group leadership by community members, and newsletters with cultural focus.	Neither group achieved weight loss. Increased levels of physical activity in both groups, but no statistically significant differences. IG had sig. increases in BMI, systolic & diastolic blood pressure & plasma conce-ntrations of glucose. CG. had sig. decreases in waist circumference & starch intake.

Table 4. (Continued)

Name of Study & Reference	Geographic Location Target Audience Sample Size	Study design & duration	Goals	Intervention	Community Involvement/ Cultural Relevance	Results
Clinical Interventions						
WISEWOMAN Heart Disease Prevention for Alaska Native Women Witmer et al., 2004	ANs and AI living in the Anchorage Service Unit Adult women ages 40-64 N=75 (total)	Pilot trial randomized into intervention group (IG) and control group (CG). 1 year	Reduce risk factors for heart disease including obesity, diet, physical activity, and tobacco use. Assess feasibility & cultural acceptability of the study & develop enrollment procedures.	12 weekly sessions taught by multidisciplinary team on lifestyle change & goal setting.	Intervention tailored to AN women & adapted to reflect AN culture.	No sig differences in groups for cholesterol, blood pressure or BMI. IG had sig improvement in walking frequency, physical activity self-efficacy & psychological changes. IG moved from contemplation to action stage. Findings from large scale study not yet available.
Community-Based Interventions						
Stop Diabetes! Marlow et al., 1998	Winnebago Tribe in Nebraska Adolescents ages 13-18 N=24	Quasi-experimental. One-group, pre-posttest design. Pilot study. Summer 1995	Diabetes prevention including physical activity, nutrition, & information provided within a cultural context.	Educational half-day workshop that included traditional games, food preparation, measurement of BMI & body fat, individual fitness profile, & manual.	Native American stories provided cultural framework. AI adolescents involved in 8 planning meetings & led other participants by example.	9 pre/post knowledge questionnaires completed; mean pretest score 49%, mean posttest score 90%. Of 10 completed evaluations, 9 reported a positive experience.

Community-Based Interventions

Name of Study & Reference	Geographic Location Target Audience Sample Size	Study design & duration	Goals	Intervention	Community Involvement/ Cultural Relevance	Results
Zuni Diabetes Project: Weight Loss Competition Health et al., 1991	Zuni and Pine Hill communities of Southwest New Mexico Adults men & women N=271	Quasi-experimental, one group pre-posttest design. 10 weeks	Weight loss of 2.3 kg for 10 weeks	Part of a statewide nutrition education and weight control program. Educational packet. New message/ behaviors assigned every 2 weeks & reinforced on TV. Incentives offered for participation & goal achievement. Weekly weigh-in sessions available & exercise logs provided.	Community teams of 35-50 persons participated. Team weight loss posted in community locations.	Finishers included goal-weight achievers (N=122) & non-goal weight achievers (N=126). Achievers significantly more likely to be male, to maintain exercise log, & to be women who had greater initial weight. Achievers also changed eating behaviors (e.g., more veggies, less ice cream).
Cultural Health and Mobilization Project (CHAMP) Pargee et al., 1999	7 rural & urban communities of AIs in northern California: Smith River, Weitchpec, Crescent City, Klamath, Arcata /McKinley-ville, ureka/Fortuna & Pecwan. Families including elders N=605	Qualitative assessment 3 year grant	Increase physical activity levels among 20 % of tribal population. Increase knowledge & change attitudes towards physical activity in order to reduce incidence of diabetes &	Community coalitions were established. Coalitions planned local events for families; for example, stick games, surf fishing, community gardening, sports tournaments, family fitness nights. Coalitions facilitated by health promotion staff. A core coalition with reps from each of	Prevention framework based on traditional Native values. Native Americans from each region hired as health promotion staff. Residents invited to attend monthly forums to plan their communities' fitness activities.	Not all community coalition efforts were successful, but several of the coalition activities were institutionalized as annual events. Success facilitated by coalition member participation, skill mastery by active participation, and inclusion of all generations. Specific outcomes not reported.

Table 4. (Continued)

Name of Study & Reference	Geographic Location Target Audience Sample Size	Study design & duration	Goals	Intervention	Community Involvement/ Cultural Relevance	Results
Clinical Interventions						
			cardiovascular disease.	coalitions met quarterly.		
The Diabetes Wellness Project Struthers et al., 2003 Washington Post, 2002 Seva Foundation	Winnebago Reservation in Nebraska & Oglala Lakota Pine Ridge Reservation in South Dakota AIs with and without a diagnosis of diabetes N-147	Quasi-experimental. Intervention group (IG) & comparison group (CG) 1998-2002	Education about diabetes management & treatment & diabetes prevention, including obesity prevention.	IG: Community gathering involving 12 weekly sessions led by trained community facilitators. Participants tell stories, convey information, express concerns, & reach decisions. CG: received usual diabetes care & health education.	Talking Circles used as a way to integrate Native American's oral traditions, storytelling, and Western medical information. Tribal members served as facilitators of the Circles	No difference between IG & CG on BMI. Sig decrease in fatalistic attitudes among at risk cohort in IG. Sig increase in knowledge in IG vs. CG.
Pathways Caballero et al., 2003 Gittlesohn et al., 2003 Steckler et al., 2003 Davis et al., 2003	AI children living in Arizona, New Mexico & South Dakota Children from 41 schools in 3rd-5th grades N=1,704	Randomized controlled trial 1993-1996	Evaluate the effectiveness of a school-based multi-component intervention for reducing percentage of body fat in AI schoolchildren.	School-based intervention involving dietary intake in school setting, physical activity in schools, classroom curriculum focused on lifestyle & nutrition, & family involvement.	Cultural concepts & traditions integrated into the curriculum by use of stories, games, music, art work, foods, family activities, & videos.	No sig reduction in body fat between IG and CG schools, but significant reduction in % of energy from fat in IG schools. No significant differences in physical activity, but significant changes in knowledge, attitudes and behaviors.

Clinical Interventions

Name of Study & Reference	Geographic Location Target Audience Sample Size	Study design & duration	Goals	Intervention	Community Involvement/ Cultural Relevance	Results
Southwest Cardiovascular Curriculum Project Davis et al., (1995)	Navaho & Pueblo children at or near reservations in rural NM 5th graders from 11 schools N=2,018	Quasi-experimental pretest posttest design with intervention (IG) and control group (CG) schools 1988-1993	Promote cardiovascular health and behavior change.	IGMulti-disciplinary school-based program with 2 hour/week curriculum over 13 weeks focusing on exercise, nutrition, tobacco, & social influences. CG intervention activities phased in during Years 4& 5.	Elders used as teachers to discuss traditions. Students interviewed their family members about exercise & diet. Lessons included AI legacy of running & active games & traditional diet.	IG showed sig increases in knowledge and exercise & used salt and butter significantly less often than CG.
Zuni Diabetes Prevention Program Tuefel & Ritenbaugh, 1998	Zuni adolescents in Arizona 9-12th grade high school students N=119-173	Quasi-experimental. Multiple cross-sectional model. Baseline characteristics of sample compared with Anglo youth of same age living in Tucson. 4 years.	Reduce prevalence of diabetes risk factors among high-school-age adolescents. Includes focus on knowledge, attitudes and beliefs about food choices and physical activity.	School-based intervention involving diabetes education, school-based wellness center, supportive social networks, & modification of the food supply available to teens.	Efforts made to develop community, faculty and youth supportive social networks. Peers employed as health advisors	Over time, Zuni youths sig. decreased their beverage consumption and had a decline in incidence of hyperinsulinemia. Non-sig. findings indicate behaviors changed in line with goals of study.
Tsitewatakari: tat Let's Get Healthy Hood et al., 1997 IHS, 2000	Akwesasne Tribe in New York Pre-K to 6th grade youth No information on N	Quasi-experimental study. No comparison group. 1993-1998	Prevention of obesity and diabetes. Reduce dietary fat and increase physical	School-based primary prevention program involving a curriculum, community exercise classes,	Pilot study prior to this study involved formation of comm-unity coalition that initiated wellness programs.	In 1994, more than 50 % of children were overweight, and in 1998, 90 % were overweight. A healthy lifestyle was not

Table 4. (Continued)

Clinical Interventions						
Name of Study & Reference	**Geographic Location Target Audience Sample Size**	**Study design & duration**	**Goals**	**Intervention**	**Community Involvement/ Cultural Relevance**	**Results**
			activity in young children.	diabetes education in-services, teacher interviews, & body fat measurements.		achieved for at least half of the children.
Kahnawake Schools Diabetes Prevention Paradis et al., 2005	Mohawk children in Canada Children 6-11 years of age N=410 (IG) & 200 (CG)	Quasi-experimental. Mixed cross-sectional & longitudinal design with a nonequivalent comparison group of children. 8 years	Prevention of diabetes including reduction of obesity, high calorie & high fat diet & physical inactivity.	Community-based program including health education in grades 1-6; community activities; collaboration with community agencies; training of Native staff, volunteers & community members; environmental & policy changes.	Participatory research, community ownership & grassroots participation at all levels of planning, delivery & evaluation.	Early outcome results that showed some success in reducing risk factors for type 2 diabetes, but were not maintained over 8 years. Process evaluation found increases in healthy food choices at school, classroom diabetes prevention activities, & ecological changes e.g., improvements in school nutrition policy & community walking path.
Pilot Home Visiting Study Harvey-Berino & Rourke, 2003	St. Regis Mohawk community of Akwesasne in northern New York State, Ontario & Quebec, Canada.	Random assignment to Intervention Group (IG) & and Comparison Group	Determine if IG - maternal participation in the obesity prevention plus parenting	Parents assigned to obesity prevention plus parenting support (IG) or parenting support (CG). Both had 16 week home-	Indigenous peer educator conducted intervention.	Children's weight-for-height scores were not sig, but showed a trend towards sig, decreasing in the IG and increasing in the CG. IG children

Clinical Interventions						
Name of Study & Reference	**Geographic Location Target Audience Sample Size**	**Study design & duration**	**Goals**	**Intervention**	**Community Involvement/ Cultural Relevance**	**Results**
	Family had child between 9 months-3 years, child was walking, mother's BMI over 25 kg/m2,	(CG). Pilot study.	support intervention would reduce prevalence of obesity in high risk	based program conducted by peer educator. In IG,		sig decreased energy intake.
	mother agreed to treatment appointments. N=43 mother-child pairs	16 week intervention	children when compared to a parenting support-only intervention. - CG	educator focused on parenting skills around eating and exercise in children, but refrained from discussing these issues in CG.		Mothers in IG used less restrictive feeding practices over time. Body weight & BMI decreased for mothers, but changes not significant over time or between groups.

The process of using ecological strategies involves consensus building and community involvement, and an ecological model is consistent with Native American beliefs that an individual's health and well-being is interrelated to the health of the family, community and environment (Smedley & Syme).

Story et al. (2003) point out that several aspects of the environment of low-income American Indian communities are important in considering the problem of obesity. These environments need improved access to healthier food choices; safe, affordable physical activity opportunities such as neighborhood centers with facilities for physical activity; community recreation programs; playgrounds with adequate equipment; and community trails for hiking, biking and physical fitness.

Both clinical and community-based approaches are likely to be required for the goals of preventing or delaying obesity/diabetes. Intervention studies in both categories are reviewed in this section.

Clinical Interventions

The Diabetes Prevention Program (DPP). The DPP was a 27-center randomized clinical trial funded by multiple components of the NIH, with the National Institute of Diabetes and Digestive and Kidney Diseases (NIDDK) as the lead institute. This important study occurred between 1996-2001 and included AI/ANs among other groups. The purpose of the study was to determine whether lifestyle intervention or pharmacological therapy (metformin) would prevent or delay the onset of diabetes in individuals with impaired glucose tolerance (IGT) who are at high risk for the disease (DPP Research Group, 2000a).

There were 3,235 participants in the study; approximately half of them were from racial or ethnic minority groups including American Indians, African Americans, Asian Americans and Pacific Islanders, and Hispanic Americans. Five percent (N=171) of the participants were American Indian from urban and reservation communities in the Southwest including the Salt River, Zuni, Gila River Indian Community and Navajo Tribes. The mean age of all participants was 51 years, the mean BMI was 34, and sixty-eight percent of the total sample were women.

Participants were randomly assigned to one of three interventions:

- Standard lifestyle recommendations (e.g., written information and an annual individual session) plus metformin;
- Standard lifestyle recommendations plus placebo; or
- Intensive program of lifestyle modification entitled Lifestyle Balance.

Findings indicated no significant difference in treatment effects by racial or ethnic group or by sex; thus, findings regarding the incidence of diabetes for American Indians participants did not differ from those of other groups in the study (see Exhibit 1). Results indicated that the lifestyle intervention reduced the incidence of diabetes by 58% and metformin by 31%, as compared with placebo; the lifestyle intervention was significantly more effective than metformin in reducing the incidence of diabetes (DPP Research Group, 2000a) (see Exhibit 2). Participants assigned to the lifestyle intervention had significantly greater weight loss (see Exhibit 3) and a greater increase in leisure physical activity than did participants in the other two groups. The average follow-up period was 2.8 years. Study results supported the hypothesis that type 2 diabetes can be prevented or delayed in persons at high risk for the disease. The blinded treatment phase was terminated 1 year early in May 2001 because the data had clearly answered the main research questions.

The intensive lifestyle intervention had a similar goal for all participants -- a 7% weight loss and at least 150 minutes of physical activity per week. A 16-lesson curriculum covering diet, exercise and behavior modification was designed to help participants achieve these goals (DPP Research Group, 2000b). Lifestyle coaches from same ethnic group as the participants taught the curriculum on a one-to-one basis during the first 24 weeks of enrollment. Subsequent individual (usually monthly) and group sessions with the lifestyle coaches were designed to reinforce behavioral changes. The key aspects of the intensive Lifestyle Balance intervention were as follows:

- A goal-based behavioral intervention;
- Case managers or "lifestyle coaches" often chosen from the same ethnic group as the participant to deliver the intervention;
- Frequent contact and ongoing intervention throughout the trial to help participants achieve and maintain weight and physical activity goals;
- "Toolbox" strategies that tailored the intervention to the individual participant;
- Intervention materials and strategies to address the needs of an ethnically diverse population; for example, information about foods and cooking methods used by various ethnic groups, cooking classes with familiar foods, or simplified self-monitoring forms; and
- An intensive local and national network that provided training, feedback and clinical support for the interventionists.

A follow-up clinical study to the DPP entitled the *Diabetes Prevention Program Outcomes Study (DPPOS*) is currently being conducted by NIDDK, and is described in detail in the NIH section of this report. Similarly to the DPP, this study includes a sample of AIs as well as other racial and ethnic groups.

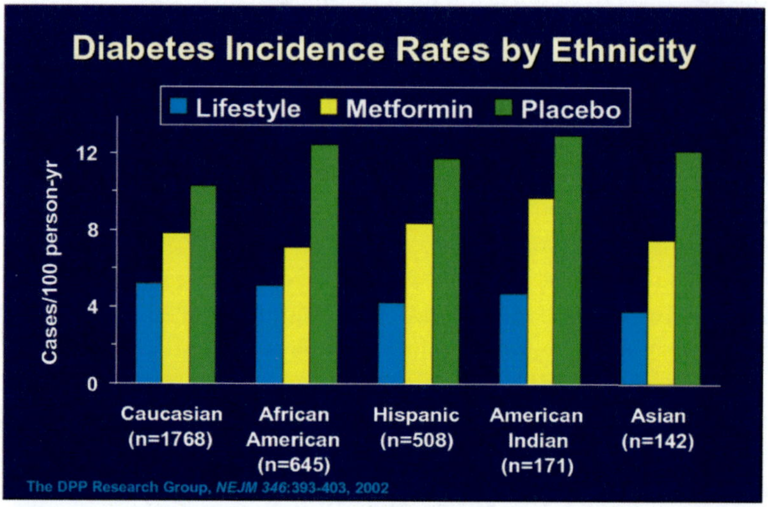

Exhibit 1.

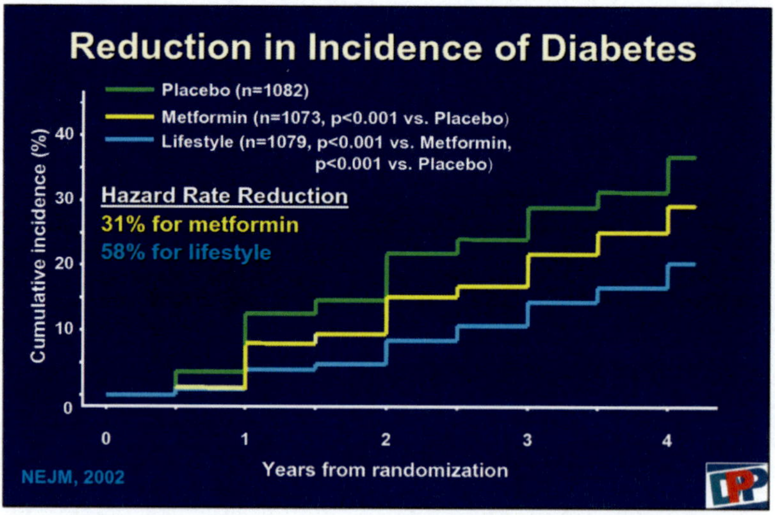

Exhibit 2.

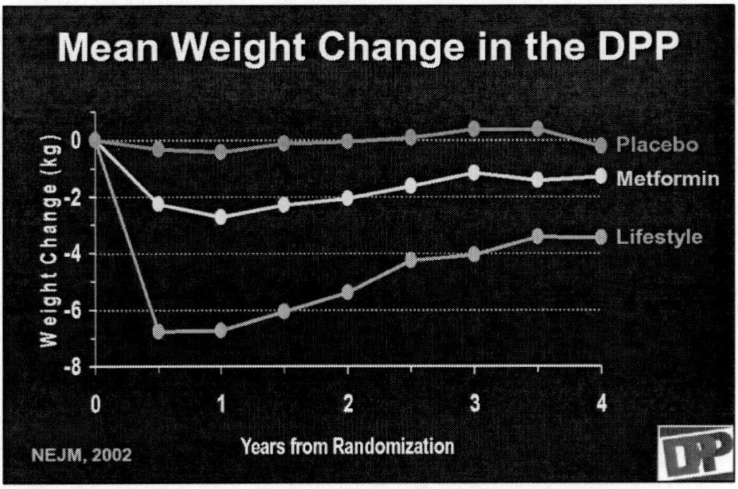

Exhibit 3.

Lifestyle Interventions in Pima Indians: a Pilot Study. A pilot trial was conducted to test adherence to specific lifestyle interventions among Pima Indians of Arizona. Ninety-five obese men and women age 25-54 years were randomized to treatments -- Pima Action (Action) and Pima Pride (Pride) which were tested for 12 months (Narayan et al., 1998).

The Action group (N=47) involved structured activity and nutrition interventions including opportunities for physical activities, weekly group meetings, home visits as appropriate, behavioral techniques, role-playing, group problem-solving, food preparation demonstrations, food tasting, and grocery store tours. The Pride intervention (N=48) focused on unstructured activities that emphasized Pima history and culture including monthly groups that discussed attitudes and lifestyles of the community and included local speakers on Pima culture and history. Pride participants also received written information on healthy eating and exercise habits. In both groups, adherence to interventions, changes in self-reported activity and diet, and changes in weight, glucose concentrations, and other risk factors were assessed regularly.

Reported physical activity of both groups increased; however there were no significant differences in outcomes between the two groups. The Pride group had a greater decrease in energy, starch, carbohydrate, and fat intake than members of the Action group, but these differences were also not significant. After 1 year, weight, BMI, systolic blood pressure, diastolic blood pressure, 2-h glucose, 2-h insulin had all increased significantly in the Action group, and waist circumference had decreased significantly in the Pride group.

Members of the Action group gained more weight on average than the Pride group, but this difference also was not significant. Thus, the Pride intervention emphasizing self-directed learning and culture was more effective at preventing weight gain and glucose intolerance than the Action intervention using structured activity and nutrition education, *but neither intervention achieved weight loss on average.* The researchers stated that weight loss among people at risk for type 2 diabetes is difficult and sustaining adherence to behavior interventions was challenging; attendance at nutrition classes declined over time.

The changes in activity levels and diet among the Pride group were not understood because these factors were not directly emphasized in the Pride group. The researchers speculated that lifestyle interventions using direct methods to target specific risk factors (e.g., diet and activity) may not be compatible with Native American values and indirect, unstructured and participatory approaches may be more successful in some groups. The authors hypothesized that the emphasis on self-directed learning through an appreciation of Pima culture may have empowered the Pride individuals toward a healthier lifestyle, but they also said that simply being in a trial or having measurements taken may have prompted action. Furthermore, they hypothesized that the main determinant of the Pride group's success may have been social support, but this variable was not measured.

The researchers concluded that future lifestyle intervention studies need to take further account of local culture and values and more effectively address potential constraints to participation such as patient preference and socioeconomic factors (e.g., lack of transportation, need for child care, alcohol-related problems, and other social factors). Although participants said they wanted weekly classes, this schedule may have been too onerous, and researchers thought that less frequent but more intensive sessions may be more successful. They noted that while the interventions significantly increased physical activity levels within groups, modification of dietary factors was less successful. They found that many of the participants compensated for reducing the fat in their diet by increasing the total intake of foods, particularly low fat items. Thus they recommended that the nutrition component should emphasize total calorie reduction, weight loss, and weight-monitoring in addition to reduction in dietary fat. The researchers suggested that lifestyle interventions may be more effective in some populations if they were delivered to randomized family units rather than to individuals.

WISEWOMAN Heart Disease Prevention for Alaska Native (AN) Women. The SouthCentral Foundation, an AN-owned health corporation, conducted a pilot randomized controlled trial of a heart disease prevention program tailored for Alaska native women (Witmer et al., 2004). The study was carried out as part of the Well-integrated Screening and Evaluation for Women Across the Nation (WISEWOMAN) Program funded by CDC (See CDC section of this report for full description of this program). The aim of the pilot was to assess the feasibility and cultural acceptability of the study and to develop enrollment procedures. The small sample included 75 women ages 40-64 who lived within 50 miles of Anchorage, were due for an annual Pap test, and had selected one of the four participating physicians as their primary care practitioner. Forty- four of the women were randomized to the intervention group and 32 to the control group (i.e., delayed intervention). The intervention was adapted to reflect AN culture and included 12 weekly sessions taught by a multidisciplinary team on lifestyle change (e.g., nutrition, physical activity, and tobacco use) and goal setting. At baseline and 12 months, participant's height, weight, resting blood pressure, fasting lipid levels, and blood glucose were measured. Additionally, responses of the intervention group to pre- and posttest questionnaires at sessions 1 and 12 were compared in regard to diet, physical activity, tobacco use, and psychosocial status.

At 12 months, no significant differences were found between the two groups for cholesterol, blood pressure, or BMI. While the small sample size precluded drawing conclusions about the intervention's effect, significant improvements were noted among the intervention participants in moderate walking frequency; physical activity self-efficacy (i.e., confidence in ability to achieve regular physical activity); and psychosocial changes such as being more likely to ask family and friends for support, less stress-induced eating, and a greater likelihood of working off stress using physical activity. Also, in the intervention group, there was substantial movement from the contemplation and preparation stages to the action stage regarding physical activity and heart-healthy eating. This pilot study resulted in protocol changes that improved the design and implementation of a subsequent large scale study; findings are not yet available from this study.

Community-Based Interventions

Stop Diabetes! An Educational Model for Native American Adolescents in the Prevention of Diabetes. This pilot one-group pretest/post test intervention was designed by four Winnebago adolescents for their peers residing on their Nebraska reservation (N=24) and carried out during the summer of 1995. The intervention was educational in nature, focusing on diabetes prevention through physical activity and good nutrition within a cultural context understandable to these adolescents (Marlow et al., 1998).

Four adolescents, self-named the Coyotes, assisted in the development and leadership of this program during eight weekly planning meetings. The image of the Coyote in Native American legend symbolizes the concept of indirect education or teaching by example. The Coyotes, by their example, indirectly led other adolescents and reflected the cultural aspects of this program.

The curriculum included information about diabetes, physical activity, and nutrition. Native American stories and legends provided the cultural framework for discussing the healthful aspects of traditional AI life. Participation involved attending a half-day workshop which included traditional games; preparation of nutritious foods; measurement of BMI, body fat, fat- free mass, and total body water; an individualized fitness profile; and a student manual. Participants were asked to complete pre and post-workshop knowledge questionnaires and a workshop evaluation form.

Only 9 of 24 sets of pre-post workshop knowledge questionnaires were completed. The mean score for these pretests was 49 percent, while the mean posttest score was 90 percent. And, of the 10 completed evaluations of the study, 9 indicated a positive workshop experience.

The researchers recommended that future programs be grounded in the Native American worldview which is a holistic, pluralistic perspective that emphasizes group work and cooperation. This is in contrast to the linear, individualistic and competitive focus of the Western worldview that is used in many health education materials for Native Americans. In developing future projects, Marlow et al., recommended: 1) establishing links with a broad spectrum of community resources; 2) including an adolescent advisory group that meets regularly with adults to plan and monitor programs; and 3) developing health education materials and data collection instruments that reflect Native American learning styles and traditional culture.

Zuni Diabetes Project: Weight-Loss Competition. A 10-week community-wide weight-loss competition was held in conjunction with the "Eat Right New Mexico" campaign – a statewide nutrition education and weight-control program. Participants were from the Zuni and Pine Hill communities in Southwest New Mexico. They paid a $5.00 registration fee and provided basic demographic information including their weight.

They received an educational packet consisting of five nutrition and health messages. A new message and set of behaviors were assigned every 2 weeks and were reinforced by statewide television. The weight-loss goal was 2.3 kg for the 10 weeks of participation. Incentives were offered for different levels of participation and levels of goal achievement. Teams of 35-50 members were composed of individuals sharing affiliations with a worksite, exercise group, or specific community. Weekly weigh-in sessions were available by coordinators at six team sites, and exercise logs were provided with a generic prescription to perform aerobic exercise for 20 minutes or more three times per week. Total weight loss for each team was graphically illustrated on display boards that were posted in four community locations (Health et al., 1991).

This competition was evaluated by IHS. At its completion, participants were divided into three groups: those who did not complete the program (non-finishers, N=22), those who finished but did not lose 2.3 kg or more (non-goal achievers, N=126), and those who finished and lost more than 2.3 kg (goal-weight achievers, N=122). Of the 271 registered participants, 249 (92 percent) completed the program. Goal-weight achievers (45 percent of the enrollees) were significantly different from non-goal achievers in the following ways: 1) more likely to be male (77 percent of males versus 45 percent of females achieved the goal), 2) women more likely to have greater initial weight, and 3) more likely to maintain an exercise log (59 percent versus 36 percent). Four behavior changes were significantly different between the two groups: cutting down on cream and ice cream, eating unsweetened foods for breakfast, buying bread made with whole wheat, and increasing the amount of vegetables in the diet.

The researchers stated that although average weight loss was modest, this program represents one of only a few attempts to promote weight loss on a community-wide scale in AI populations. Furthermore, this type of competition is an inexpensive strategy for facilitating behavioral change in communities similar to the Zuni Indians. They speculated that social support theory may explain why such competitions may work; for example, team competitions could strengthen support by team members and, thereby, stimulate interest, increase commitment, and facilitate long-term behavioral change.

Cultural Health and Mobilization Project (CHAMP) This program involved a 3-year grant from the California Department of Health Services to implement a project that focused on promoting physical activity with AI community coalitions in seven urban and rural communities of AIs in

Northern California. The primary objectives of this program were to: 1) increase physical activity levels among 20 percent of the local tribal population, and 2) to increase knowledge and change attitudes toward physical activity in order to reduce the incidence of diabetes and cardiovascular disease (Pargee et al., 1999).

The prevention framework that was used was based on traditional Native American values including: belonging (inclusive of all ages and all people); mastery (empowerment for individuals and the community); the interdependence of action, community leadership and the environment; and the generosity of community elders who give their knowledge to future generations. This holistic approach reflects the Native American belief that the health of the individual is interdependent with the health of the family, community and environment. Furthermore, the program was built upon knowledge of AIs as group-oriented, consensus-based decision makers as well as culturally appropriate community ownership concepts.

Using key Native Americans hired from each of the regions as health promotion staff, community coalitions were established in each of the communities, and residents were invited to attend forums to discuss health problems facing each community as well as solutions. These coalitions met monthly as planning groups to design and organize their communities' fitness promotion activities, and representatives of each of the coalitions combined to form a core coalition that met quarterly.

The coalitions chose local events as a means whereby traditional knowledge could be presented in a manner that was relevant as a health education message. Activities involved whole families so that elders had a chance to teach younger generations. The community events created an environment in which individuals learned by doing. Examples of the types of traditional cultural activities carried out at these events included surf fishing, stick games, gathering of basket- making materials, making ceremonial regalia, and community gardening. Positive family activities were also a priority such as community walking groups, sports tournaments, and family fitness nights. All events were community driven and organized by the coalitions with facilitation by the health promotion staff.

Not all of the community coalition building efforts were successful; however, several of the coalition activities were institutionalized by tribal governments as annual events. Community support was most successful in areas in which the coalitions could build on previously successful community events. Challenges arose when key people who had been involved in previous community activities dropped out of the coalition due to overwhelming responsibilities, and as a result, attendance at coalition meetings declined. Furthermore, initially, coalitions did not have clarity of purpose; thus, the staff had to learn to delegate authority to community members and to facilitate the coalitions, and this trust-building process was time-consuming. Although specific outcomes on physical activity levels, attitudes or knowledge were not reported, the authors concluded that active planning and participation by coalition members, including all generations in activities, ensuring mastery of skills by active participation, and drawing on the wisdom of elders to teach younger generations helped make the coalitions successful. The authors stated that, "The influence of culture on health acts as a positive force; joining communities to promote community wellness, weaving cultural wisdom into health promotion."

The Diabetes Wellness Project. The overall goal of this project was to reduce the mortality and morbidity of type 2 diabetes among adult AIs by improving prevention practices and diabetic treatment compliance. Funded by the National Institutes of Nursing Research and the Centers for Disease Control and Prevention, the intervention involved a culturally appropriate approach called the Talking Circles. Conducted during 1998-2003, four tribal sites were involved in this study – Winnebago Reservation, Nebraska; Porcupine Pine Ridge Reservation, South Dakota; Rosebud Reservation, South Dakota; and Yankton Reservation, South Dakota - and these sites were randomized into intervention and control sites. A total of 324 persons participated in this study—147 in the intervention group and 177 in the control group.

Talking Circles involve a community gathering where participants tell stories, convey information, express concerns, and reach decisions. In the two intervention tribes, twelve weekly sessions were conducted by trained community facilitators who provided information on the prevention and management of diabetes, including obesity prevention. Participants included those who have a diagnosis of diabetes as well as those who are at risk of diabetes. The two control tribes received usual diabetes care and health education (Struthers et al., 2003).

The Talking Circle format has been used for health education and promotion and provides a way to integrate Native American oral traditions, storytelling and Western medical information (Hodge et al., 2002). During the Talking Circles, participants numbered between 5 and 20. They sat in chairs placed in a circle. The community facilitators were key to the project; they recruited the participants, held them in the circle, and provided skillful guidance in a comfortable, supportive and confidential setting. There was an important spiritual component to the intervention; the session stared with a participant offering a prayer to the Creator and a traditional/teaching story specific to the tribe. The facilitator then presented information on diabetes and obesity prevention topics from the curriculum. Each participant was given the opportunity to speak and many told stories about their experiences. When speaking, a participant may hold a feather, rock or other symbolic item. After each person has had a chance to contribute, the facilitator summarizes the events, and the Talking Circle is closed.

During the first session, weight and other physical measurements were taken as well as a self- administered pretest, and at the concluding session, these measurements were retaken along with a posttest. Additionally, with participant knowledge and informed consent, research staff reviewed clinic health charts of the Talking Circle participants for specific data.

While there was no difference in BMI measurements between the intervention and control groups, an analysis of the other group differences indicated two main findings: (Hodge, 2007).

- Prior to their involvement in the study, participants held fatalistic attitudes regarding prevention, onset and control of diabetes. Following the intervention, post-test scores indicated there was a significant decrease in fatalism among the "at risk" cohort (i.e. those who were at risk for diabetes, but did not yet have this condition) in the intervention group when compared to the control group.
- Participants significantly increased their diabetes knowledge scores following the intervention, when compared with the control group. Total knowledge consisted of information pertaining to diabetes, fiber food, fatty food, and exercise. Increase in total knowledge for the intervention group was significant for both men and women and for diabetics as well as for those "at risk." Multiple regression analysis also indicated that the increase in knowledge for the intervention group was significantly greater than for the control group.

In a subsequent qualitative substudy conducted after the intervention, the researchers interviewed 8 participants who had attended all 12 sessions about their experiences in the Talking Circle. The interviewees ranged in age from 40-70; 5 were female and 5 had diabetes. Analysis of responses revealed seven common themes: (1) the effect of living with diabetes in the community and in their families; 2) the need to express the loss, sadness and grief the disease had caused; 3) the worth of receiving current information about diabetes in a setting where they could understand and discuss it; 4) the importance of sharing their stories and experiences; 5) the value of obtaining guidance from the facilitator who lived in their community; 6) the need to incorporate diabetes information with their traditional practices and beliefs; and 7) the need to take action, individually, within their family, and within their tribes, to spread information about diabetes and to help prevent or slow its occurrence. Researchers concluded that the Talking Circles provided an effective and culturally appropriate forum for members of these tribal communities to learn about diabetes and help spread information about proper management and treatment to others (Struthers et al., 2003a).

The Indian Health Service has adopted the Talking Circle model as a Best practice (IHS, 2006). Talking Circle facilitators have been trained at tribal sites in Nebraska, South Dakota, North Dakota, New Mexico, Montana, and Wyoming, and training is ongoing for tribes in Minnesota, Michigan and Wisconsin. Training for other interested tribes will be offered at IHS' 2007 Summer Institute in Albuquerque (De Cora, 2006; Seva Foundation, 2006). Support for the online tutorial materials is being provided by the Seva Foundation, CDC's Native Diabetes Wellness Program and the Robert Wood Johnson Community Leadership Program.

Pathways. This 3-year study initiated in 1993 was a school-based multicomponent intervention for the prevention of obesity in AI school children supported by the National Heart, Lung and Blood Institute (NHLBI). The study was a randomized controlled trial involving 1,704 3rd-5th grade obese and nonobese AI children in 41 schools in Arizona, New Mexico and South Dakota. The four components of the study included: change in dietary intake in the school setting; 2) increase in physical activity in the school setting; 3) classroom curriculum focused on health eating and lifestyle; and 4) family involvement. Cultural concepts and traditions were integrated into the curriculum through the use of stories, games, music, art work, foods, family activities and videos.

The intervention resulted in no significant reduction in percentage of body fat; however, there was a significant reduction in the percentage of energy from fat consumed at meals in the schools. Furthermore, there were no significant differences found in physical activity between the intervention and control schools. However, there were significant and positive changes that occurred with regard to knowledge, attitudes and behaviors; for example, increased consumption of fruits and vegetables, fewer calories from fat, increased physical activity while at school, greater weight-related knowledge, heightened ethnic identity, and reduced TV watching. Finally, there was a significant retention of knowledge over the 3 years for the intervention group.

The researchers concluded that interventions may need to start earlier and last longer and may need to address a broader range of factors that influence caloric intake and physical activity such as environmental and socioeconomic factors beyond the school setting. They indicated that they knew very little about what the children did after they left school, and that this was a large gap in this study. They concluded that there was a need for further research on family processes and behavior and for better methods to measure the effectiveness of family interventions. The researchers suggested outreach to families in settings other than schools; for example local fairs, pow wows, and grocery stores (Caballero et al., 2003; Gittelsohn et al., 2003; Steckler et al., 2003; Davis et al., 2003).

Southwest Cardiovascular Curriculum Project. From 1988-1993, a school-based program to promote cardiovascular health behavior change was conducted for 5th grade Navajo and Pueblo students at 11 elementary schools located at or near Indian reservations in rural New Mexico (N=2,018). Participating schools were randomly assigned to intervention versus control groups. The intervention included a 2 hour/week curriculum over the course of 13 weeks that focused on exercise, nutrition, tobacco, and social influences. The control schools did not receive the curriculum during the first 3 years of the study and were phased in at the community's request during the final 2 years. Pre and posttests were used with both groups to measure health knowledge, attitudes and self-reported behaviors.

The program was designed to incorporate Native traditions and values. Elders were used as teachers to discuss the importance of traditions, and students interviewed their own family members about their eating and exercise habits when they were growing up. Lessons on fitness and nutrition incorporated the Native Americans' legacy of running and active games and a diet that included red and green chiles, corn, beans, and squash.

Study findings indicated that students in the intervention group showed significant increases in knowledge when compared with controls for both Navajos and Pueblos. A significantly higher proportion of students in the intervention group reported a decrease in the frequency of salt use at the table and butter use on bread tortillas. Seventy percent of students in the intervention group reported increasing the amount they exercised since baseline, compared to 55 percent in the control group. Overall Navajo schools showed more positive significant differences than did the Pueblos in response to the curriculum.

Researchers concluded that a primary prevention program utilizing a culturally-oriented curriculum is one approach that can be effective in promoting healthful lifestyles in an AI population (Davis et al., 1995).

Zuni Diabetes Prevention Program. This school-based program was conducted with Zuni 9th-12th grade high school students in Arizona (N=119 at Year 1; 173 at Year 3) over a 4 year period. The purpose was to target non-insulin dependent type 2 diabetes risk factors including obesity; insulin resistance; physical activity levels; consumption of sugared beverages and high-fiber foods; and knowledge, attitudes and beliefs about this condition, food choices, and physical activity.

The intervention consisted of: 1) the establishment of supportive social networks (e.g., community, faculty and youth); 2) construction of a wellness facility designed for teens; 3) diabetes education integrated with the classroom curriculum; and 4) modification of the food supply available to teens (e.g., vending machine snacks and meals). At the onset of the program, no sugar-free beverages were available in the vending machines. In years 1 and 2, sugar-free selections were added, and in years 3 and 4, only sugar-free selections were available. The Zuni adolescents were compared to Anglo youngsters of the same age residing in Tucson on baseline characteristics including height, weight, fasting and insulin/glucose values.

Over the course of 2 years, Zuni youth had decreased their BMI, decreased consumption of sugared beverages, increased consumption of dietary fiber, decreased sitting pulse rates (e.g., improved cardiovascular fitness), and increased glucose/insulin ratios (e.g., decline in hyperinsulinemia); however, only the changes in the beverage consumption and insulin levels were significant over time.

The researchers concluded that the degree to which health promotion activities can alter a school's routine and curricula depend on the flexibility of the faculty and administrators and the integration of the health promotion effort within the curriculum. Interestingly, they also characterized this intervention as ubiquitous versus directive, as it provided cues that health promotion as a gentle and consistent part of the students' lives (e.g., occasional classroom exercises, non-sugared soft drinks in vending machines, availability of recreational equipment and activities, peers employed as health advisors) and concluded that youth behaviors were changing in a direction commensurate with the goals of the project (Tuefel & Ritenbaugh, 1998).

Tsitewatakari:tat "Let's Get Healthy" Program. This initiative involving the Mohawk People of Akwesase in New York began with a 1990-1991 pilot study (Hood et al., 1997) that resulted in the formation of a community coalition that subsequently initiated programs to reduce dietary fat and increase physical activity in young children. From 1993-1998, using funds from NIDDK, the tribe and University of Vermont health scientists began a school-based primary prevention program for obesity and diabetes with pre-K to Grade 6 children and a community-based intervention. The initiative included a comprehensive range of interventions: a curriculum, community exercise classes, diabetes education in-services, teacher interviews, and body fat measurements. At the start of the program in 1994, more than 40 percent of children were overweight, and at the end of the program in 1998, 90 percent of those children continued to be overweight (10 percent became less and 18 percent became more overweight). The investigators concluded that a healthy lifestyle involving a balanced diet and physical activity had not been achieved for at least half of the children in Akwesasne. In 1998, the program was expanded to a community and clinic-based intervention for people with or at high risk for type 2 diabetes, using funds from IHS' Special Diabetes Grants for Indians (IHS, 2001)

Kahnawake Schools Diabetes Prevention. Although this intervention was conducted with a Native population in Canada, it is included in this report because it utilized a longitudinal design over a period of 8 years and focused on obesity as well as diabetes (Paradis et al., 2005). The intervention targeted body size, physical activity and diet among Mohawk children 6-11 years of age (N=410 in the intervention group and 200 in the comparison group).

The outcome evaluation used a mixed cross-sectional and longitudinal design with a nonequivalent comparison group of children. Methods included follow-up of subjects in the intervention and comparison groups from 1994-1996 and repeat cross-sectional measurements in the intervention community alone from 1994-2002.

The implementation of this study included participatory research, community ownership and grassroots participation at all levels of planning, delivery and evaluation. The main program components included: 1) a health education curriculum delivered in grades 1-6; 2) community activities and collaborations with community agencies; 3) training of Native staff, volunteers and community members; and 4) environmental and policy changes (e.g., ban on junk foods on school premises, construction of walking and cycling path in the community).

The primary objective to reduce obesity was not achieved. Longitudinal data from 1994-1996 showed some early positive effects of the program on skinfold thickness, but not on BMI, physical activity, fitness, or diet. Repeat cross-sectional measures from 1994-2002 showed increases in skinfold thickness and BMI. Physical activity, fitness and television watching showed favorable trends from 1994 to 1999 that were not sustained in 2002. Key high-fat and high-sugar food consumption decreased, as did consumption of fruits and vegetables. Although early results showed some success in reducing risk factors for type 2 diabetes, these benefits were not maintained over 8 years. These findings suggest that earlier intervention may be indicated for those children who are overweight by the time they reach elementary school.

The process evaluation indicated increases in healthy food choices at school, classroom diabetes- prevention activities, and ecological changes such as improvements in the school nutrition policy and the community walking path, as well as strong community agreement with project objectives.

In a series of local meetings, residents suggested explanations for the increase in adiposity including: increase in community wealth and disposable income over the past decade, increased availability of fast-food restaurants in areas surrounding the reservation, increased proportion of families in which both parents work resulting in less supervision of meals and leisure activities, and the perceived importance within the community of computer literacy for youth. The researchers also speculated that television advertising could be a factor in the decreased fruit and vegetable consumption, as exposure to this type of advertising has been shown to negatively influence children's identification of healthy food choices (Signorielli & Staples, 1997).

Paradis et al., point out that societal trends over time resulting in increasing obesity throughout North America are strong and may require more intense and comprehensive efforts than a single local health promotion program. They indicate that their findings are similar to other primary prevention intervention targeting diet and physical activity among children that also have not resulted in significant reduction in average body weight or adiposity (Luepker et al., 1996; Caballero et al., 2003; Nader et al., 1999), with the exception of one study reporting significant reductions in obesity for girls only (Gortmaker et al., 1999). At the same time, these studies have been successful in achieving positive changes in diet, diet and television watching, and diet and physical activity. They also point out that the true randomized experiments have also failed to find strong unequivocal evidence of a preventive impact (Wilson et al., 2003). These researchers note that policy and environmental changes and behavior modifications for nutrition and physical activity at a community-wide level are difficult to achieve in the short term in real-life situations, because they are influenced by a complex web of very strong and pervasive social, cultural and political factors that act at numerous societal levels and are often beyond the control of a local program; for example, children are exposed to an estimated 20,000-40,000 food commercials annually, and these commercials tend to promote food high in fat and sugar by using aggressive marketing strategies.

Pilot Home Visiting Study. A pilot study using home visiting with mothers and preschool children was conducted with 43 mother-child pairs from the St. Regis Mohawk community of Akwesasne in northern New York State, Ontario and Quebec, Canada. The objective of the study was to determine whether maternal participation in an obesity prevention plus parenting support (OPPS) intervention would reduce the prevalence of obesity in high-risk Native American children when compared with a parenting support (PS)-only intervention (Harvey- Berino & Rourke, 2003).

Mothers who participated had a BMI over 25 kg/m2 and a child between 9 months and 3 years who was walking. The mother-child pairs were randomly assigned to one of the two treatment groups and they participated in a 16-week home-based program conducted by an indigenous peer educator. All the mothers participated in a core parenting program. In addition, the OPPS intervention included a focus on how improved parenting skills could facilitate the development of appropriate eating and exercise behaviors in children. Baseline and weekly assessments for mother and child included height and weight, dietary intake, physical activity, parental feeding style, maternal outcome expectations, self-efficacy, and intention to change diet and exercise behaviors.

Findings indicated that body weight and BMI decreased for mothers; however, these changes were not significant over time or between groups. The children's weight-for-height scores showed a trend toward significance, with these scores increasing in the PS condition and decreasing in the OPPS group. Children in the OPPS condition significantly decreased their energy intake. Mothers in the OPPS group were also found to engage in less restrictive child feeding practices over time (e.g., control over food intake). The researchers concluded that this program showed promise for obesity prevention in high-risk Native American children and recommended a longer intervention that would allow for a greater focus on maternal lifestyle change, a larger sample size, and the inclusion of additional mediating variables.

Summary of Intervention Research Studies

Intervention research focusing on AI/ANs and obesity prevention is in its infancy; there are only a limited number of published studies. Examination of the characteristics (not mutually exclusive) of the 13 studies described above indicated that 3 were randomized controlled trials, 8 included control or comparison groups, 4 were pilot studies, 4 had very small samples, 1 included urban Indians, and 1 intervened with the family as a unit, although other studies may have involved more than one family member in a variety of activities. Additionally, 7 of the studies occurred over a period of more than 1 year, one study was conducted for 1 year, and 4 studies were implemented for 16 weeks or less. Furthermore, these interventions reflect a wide variety of approaches taking place in different settings; for example, some are very structured clinical approaches, while others are multifaceted and take place in schools or communities.

Additionally, intervention researchers have emphasized the importance of using Native traditions and values in devising intervention strategies. There are many important Native values, but some that have been mentioned in designing culturally appropriate interventions include: the importance of connectedness and collective living; mastery (i.e., empowerment for individuals and the community), interdependence of action, community leadership and the environment; generosity of community elders who give of their knowledge to future generations (Pargee et al., 1999), understanding the complex historical journey of the American Indian as a people and as a tribe (Struthers et al., 2003); and a holistic worldview whereby a person's being is comprised of four aspects: mental, physical, emotional and spiritual. In a holistic approach, the health of the individual is interdependent with the health of the family, community and environment (Pargee et al., 1999; Struthers et al., 2003).

It is the creative incorporation of these and other Native values, culture and traditions that make obesity interventions with AI/ANs unique and more likely to result in positive outcomes. The interventions described in this section have utilized various means to do this; for example, the use of traditional Talking Circles; indigenous peer educators; community coalitions; culturally integrated curricula; or the use of traditional stories, games, music artwork, foods, or family activities.

Clinical Interventions. A clinical intervention study of major importance that included AI/ANs as well as other groups was the *Diabetes Prevention Program* (DPP) that found that the Lifestyle Balance intervention was significantly more effective in reducing the incidence of diabetes and resulted in greater weight loss and increase in leisure physical activity than interventions using a placebo or the drug metformin (see NIH section of this report). The Lifestyle Balance intervention is now being used in IHS' *Targeted Demonstration Projects* (see IHS section). Furthermore, the *Diabetes Prevention Program Outcomes Study* -- a follow-up clinical intervention study using the original DPP sample (see NIH section of this report) is now underway and is exploring the long term effect of lifestyle and drug interventions on the delay of type 2 diabetes, the maintenance of weight loss, and the occurrence of cardiovascular disease and related risk factors.

The two additional clinical interventions reported on were pilots with small samples; neither of these studies found significant differences between the intervention and comparison groups on BMI. However, these studies did find improvements within groups regarding attitudes and behaviors such as increased physical activity and movement from the contemplation or preparation stages to the action stage in terms of physical activity and diet behaviors. Lessons learned from these interventions include: 1) constraints to participation (e.g., patient preference and socioeconomic factors) need to be addressed as adherence was an issue, 2) less frequent but more intensive sessions may be more workable than weekly meetings; and 3) lifestyle interventions may be more effective if delivered to randomized family units.

Community-Based Interventions. The AI/AN–focused community-based interventions that did not involve the schools all used different approaches – talking circles, coalitions, community weight-loss competitions, and an educational workshop. Although none of these approaches reported significant weight loss, they did have an impact on attitudes, knowledge, behavior change, and the institutionalization of community events that incorporated physical activity. The two studies that combined school and community approaches were conducted over 4- and 8-year periods; similarly, neither reported significant changes in youth overweight/obesity during these time periods. However, process evaluation findings from, the 8-year study indicated increases in healthy food choices at school, classroom diabetes-prevention activities, changes in the school nutrition policy, and community walking paths. Lessons learned from these interventions include: 1) holistic group-oriented approaches that integrate Native American traditions, foster sharing and cooperation, and build on the Native American value that the health of the individual is interdependent with the health of the family, community and environment are important; and 2) the societal trend over time toward increasing obesity is strong; thus, comprehensive approaches are needed.

Three of the studies focused solely on school-based interventions. Two of these studies examined changes in BMI over time and found no significant differences between the intervention and control groups. However, all three studies did find significant positive changes with regard to knowledge, attitudes and behaviors; for example, changes in beverage consumption, increased physical activity while at school, greater weight-related knowledge, or reduced TV watching. Lessons learned from these intervention studies include: 1) recognition that interventions may need to start earlier than 3rd grade; 2) research must address environmental and socioeconomic factors beyond the school setting; 3) research on family process and behavior is needed; and 4) ubiquitous (versus directive) approaches can positively impact students' behavior; for example, non-sugared soft drinks placed in vending machines and the availability of recreational equipment and activities.

Only one home-based intervention study was located; this pilot study intervened with mother- child pairs. Findings indicated that childhood obesity was not significantly reduced. Recommendations included: a longer intervention that would allow greater focus on maternal lifestyle change, a larger sample size, and measurement of mediating variables.

General Thoughts about Community-Based Research. Many community and school intervention trials targeting individuals of all races for diet and physical activity-related chronic diseases have resulted in null, small, or modest effects (Story et al., 2003). Baranowski et al. (1998) note that positive outcomes in these trials have been weak in comparison to the resources involved, including substantial funding, multiple years of intervention, large samples, use of state-of-the-art theory, sophisticated statistical models, and the expertise of leading health behavior researchers. They suggest two reasons why these interventions are not attaining the desired level of change in behavioral outcomes: (1) current theories do not fully predict behavior or behavior change and (2) interventions are not substantially effecting change in the mediating variables.

Baranowski et al., note that new directions for prevention must include ways to change the macroenvironment and thereby change eating patterns and physical activity. For example, differences in access to healthful foods and opportunities for physical activity may be among the factors related to the prevalence of obesity in low-income communities. Thus, environmentally focused and community-based research is needed to intervene with regard to these factors. Furthermore, several researchers have stated that the involvement of AIs in the design and implementation of community-based intervention programs (i.e., participatory research) is critical to program success (Baranowski et al., 1998; Satterfield et al., 2003).

In a review of lifestyle interventions to prevent type 2 diabetes, Satterfield et al. (2003) found that common study limitations included: shortness of intervention duration, large numbers of non- responders, and inability to match pre- and post-test data or to link self-reported lifestyle changes to health outcomes/indicators (e.g., BMI). Furthermore, few studies demonstrated positive outcomes in all the intermediate outcomes of interest (e.g., healthy eating behaviors and physical activity). They recommended that researchers pursue more rigorous designs to evaluate community- and population-based interventions, including pre- and posttest designs. In addition, more studies that examine *proximal outcomes* such as self-reports or measured reports of physical activity (e.g., pedometer) and weight loss, as well as clinical coutcomes (e.g., plasma glucose levels) are needed. Studies that include examination of community change indicators such as store buying patterns or the use of walking paths might also be revealing, particularly in programs that use an ecological framework.

II. Federal Agency Activities

This section of the report describes selected key activities related to obesity or obesity prevention in four federal agencies: Indian Health Service, National Institutes of Health, Centers for Disease Control and Prevention, and the U.S. Department of Agriculture. These activities include research projects as well as other types of initiatives; some of the activities are completed while others are ongoing. Key agency informants who provided the information are listed at the end of each agency section.

Indian Health Service (IHS)

The IHS activities described in this section include the following:

- IHS Report to Congress: Obesity Prevention and Control for AIs and ANs;
- IHS Internal Obesity Workgroup;
- Special Diabetes Program for Indians (SDPI);

- Healthy Children, Healthy Families and Healthy Communities Initiative (IHS Head Start)
- IHS Obesity Data;
- On the TRAIL (Together Raising Awareness for Indian Life to Diabetes Prevention);
- Body Works; and
- Tailoring Dietary Guidelines.

IHS Report to Congress: Obesity Prevention and Control for AIs and ANs. This comprehensive report reviews the magnitude of the problem, the IHS Plan to reduce the obesity epidemic among AI/ANs, guidelines for physical activity and provider/patient interactions, risks of obesity treatment, studies of dietary intake, nutrition-related intervention studies, local tribal community intervention programs, and current national program activities (IHS, 2001). The major recommendations in this report included:

- Recognize tribal governments and work collaboratively with them;
- Develop a "Healthy Weight and Physical Activity Program" for AIs and ANs to plan, implement and evaluate obesity prevention and control programs;
- Work with other government agencies to develop interventions to reduce obesity among AI/AN communities;
- Maintain or increase health care provider expertise and access to nutrition services;
- Consider implementation of "best practices" regarding obesity prevention and management in AI/AN communities;
- Support or encourage clinical behavioral research and evaluation of public health approaches in partnership with tribes by NIH, CDC and IHS to prevent and treat obesity; and
- Establish a yearlong planning period to develop a detailed plan to address the obesity epidemic in AI/AN populations.

IHS Internal Obesity Workgroup. In April 2005, an internal workgroup met in Albuquerque, New Mexico to discuss the question: "What should IHS do in the next 2 years in the Obesity/Health Weight Initiative? IHS recognized that while interventions must address excessive caloric intake and inadequate physical activity, socioeconomic, genetic, metabolic, behavioral, environmental, historical, and cultural factors must be factored into the equation.

The purpose of the workgroup was to develop achievable short and long-term goals and outline the steps needed to achieve these goals for IHS customers and partners. In July 2005, an internal draft report was written. The overall objective was to: Reduce overweight and obesity in AI/ANs by eliminating health disparities related to healthy eating and physical activity in a culturally respectful way. This group identified the following six goals in rank order:

- Enhance and create accurate usable data;
- Transform policy into action;
- Partner with tribes to build and maximize community capacity;
- Create a new organizational workforce model to improve access to quality nutrition and physical activity services;
- Enhance integrated quality care systems; and
- Leverage and strengthen partnerships to mobilize and maximize resources.

Under each of these goals, the report identifies sub-objectives and strategies/activities. The report also lists activities pertaining to obesity awareness, prevention and treatment that IHS has been involved in as well as ideas about what IHS should do in this area over the next 2 years. The report indicated that IHS planned to consult with tribes on its draft Obesity Plan/Strategy.

Special Diabetes Program for Indians (SDPI). The SDPI is a grant program, administered by the IHS Division of Diabetes Treatment and Prevention, which provides funding for diabetes prevention and treatment services at IHS, tribal, and urban Indian health programs. Now in its tenth year, the SDPI is the most comprehensive, far-reaching diabetes program ever developed for AIs and ANs, serving tribal and urban Indian communities across the U.S. Woven into all SDPI grant programs are proven diabetes treatment and prevention strategies such as patient education on diabetes self-management, elements of quality diabetes care, and culturally appropriate physical activity, nutrition, and weight management activities.

The Balanced Budget Act of 1997 initially provided $150 million to the IHS over a 5-year period (from FY 1998-2002) to establish grants for the prevention and treatment of diabetes in AI/ANs. This funding was distributed to 333 tribal, IHS and urban Indian health entities (in 35 states) using tribal consultation, a distribution formula methodology and a formal grant application process. Subsequent legislation has increased the funding for SDPI and authorized funding through FY 2008. In December 2000, Congress passed the Consolidated Appropriations Act of 2001 which provided additional funding for the SDPI, including $70 million in FY 2001, another $70 million in FY 2002, and $100 million for FY 2003, which added 1 year to the initiative. In 2002, Congress passed HR 5738, which extended the program through 2008 and increased the amount of funding to $150 million per year. These expanded resources have enabled a greater focus on diabetes prevention; approximately two-thirds of the programs have a focus on primary and secondary prevention (e.g., improvement of dietary habits and encouragement of physical activity) with the remaining activities focused on tertiary prevention (Wilson et al., 2005).

The SDPI currently includes 399 grant programs. As directed by Congress, the IHS has established the following three major components of the program:

Community-Directed Diabetes Programs

Since 1998, the IHS has provided SDPI funds to 333 IHS, tribal, and urban Indian health programs in 35 states to begin new, or enhance existing, diabetes prevention and treatment programs. Each grant program has identified its own unique needs and priorities. The SDPI enables grantees to use their funding to design and carry out interventions that best address the problem of diabetes in their communities. The vignettes below illustrate how local programs are implementing the SDPI:

- *Cherokee Nation Diabetes Prevention Program (CNDPP), Cherokee, Oklahoma.* The focus in this program is on amount of the group's weight loss rather than the weight loss of each individual in the group. By week 16 in this program's first group, this strategy had clearly paid off with a total of 320 pounds lost. Some participants called it "weight loss motivation" because they didn't want to let their team down. Participants were encouraged to know that they were not alone in their efforts, and enjoyed being successful as a group.
- *Kenaitze Indian Tribe Diabetes Prevention Program (DPP), Kenai, Alaska.* In the DPP clinic, there is a beautifully painted mural of a river that takes up an entire wall. There are also small paddles with names on them that are placed at different points along the river and small fish are hanging from each paddle. Each paddle represents a participant in the DPP, and the fish represent an achieved goal.

Participants agree that being part of a group provided the inspiration to continue to walk and make healthy life style changes. To honor the achievements of group members, family and friends gathered to walk a mile, share a healthy meal, and acknowledge their healthy lifestyle changes. Each participant was presented with a large paddle inscribed with "Lead the Way."

Competitive Demonstration Projects

In 2004, Congress directed the IHS to develop and implement a competitive grant program to prevent diabetes in high-risk individuals and to reduce cardiovascular disease risk in people who already have diabetes. These projects are designed to translate findings from scientific studies about diabetes treatment and prevention into successful diabetes program activities in the real world settings of AI and AN communities and their health care systems. These competitive grant projects, called the "*Diabetes Prevention Demonstration Project*" and the "*Healthy Heart Demonstration Project*," were launched in 66 American Indian and Alaska Native communities at the end of 2004. A description of the Gila River Indian Community's SDPI competitive program can be found in Section III of this report.

Strengthening the Diabetes Data Infrastructure

The IHS uses administrative funding from the SDPI to strengthen the diabetes data infrastructure of the Indian health system by improving diabetes surveillance and evaluation capabilities. These funds also support the development and implementation of the IHS Electronic Health Record, the electronic patient and data management system used in Indian health facilities. These activities have enabled the IHS and diabetes grant programs to expand beyond diabetes and address diabetes-related conditions such as obesity and other chronic diseases.

An interim evaluation of the SDPI completed in December 2004 on 333 of the Community- Directed Diabetes Programs documented a wide variety of short, intermediate and long term outcomes (IHS, 2004). Some of the *short term* outcomes relevant to the prevention of obesity were:

- In 2002, 70 percent of the programs reported the availability of walking and running clubs as compared with 25 percent before the SDPI;
- 66 percent of the programs reported that they had developed an adult weight management program as compared with 28 percent before the SDPI;

- 73 percent of the programs reported the availability of primary prevention programs for children and youth as compared with 19 percent before the SDPI; and
- 50 percent of the programs reported the availability of school-based healthy eating programs for children as compared with 18 percent before the SDPI.

One of the *intermediate* outcomes relevant to the prevention of obesity was that patients in the programs that established a diabetes clinic or had a registered dietitian or public health nutritionist on their diabetes team had significantly lower mean BMIs than those in programs that did not have these resources (33.2 percent vs. 34.2 percent for diabetes clinics and 33.2 percent vs. 34.6 percent for registered dietitian/public health nutritionist on local team, respectively). And, accurate baseline data for ongoing measurement of the prevalence of diabetes and diabetes mortality long term outcomes was established with the implementation of the SDPI.

The interim evaluation also identified and described 14 Best Practice Models including: *Type 2 Diabetes in Youth-Prevention and Screening* and another for *School Health-Physical Activity and Nutrition.* Finally, challenges were identified in the areas of staffing, space, access to services, clinical issues, education, behavioral issues, evaluation and data collection, and training and technical assistance. For example, in the area of behavioral issues, 28 percent of the programs reported that community members believed there was no way to avoid diabetes, and 61 percent of the programs reported that their program needed technical assistance to help clients change behavior.

Subsequent evaluation of SDPI since the interim report of 2004 has demonstrated that SDPI grant programs have implemented many other weight management tools and activities for people with diabetes or at risk for developing diabetes. These include:

- Lifestyle and behavior change interventions;
- Innovative nutrition programs, including family nutrition, traditional food, and gardening programs;
- Physical activity programs;
- Social and group support programs;
- Individualized diet programs;
- Medication use;
- Surgery; and
- Commercial weight loss programs

Many grant programs have established focused weight management activities that involve partnerships with schools, work sites, and the community. In addition, as part of the SDPI, the IHS Division of Diabetes Treatment and Prevention has facilitated the development of several new Best Practices including: 1) *Adult Weight Management and Diabetes* and 2) *Breastfeeding*. These Best Practices, based on the positive outcomes of the grant programs, outline promising weight management and breastfeeding promotion strategies that can be implemented in AI/AN communities.

Prior to the SDPI, AI/AN communities had few resources to devote to primary prevention of diabetes. The SDPI funds have provided the resources to build a much stronger diabetes infrastructure and launch diabetes prevention activities in AI/AN communities to translate promising findings.

In FY 2004, in response to Congressional direction, competitive *Targeted Demonstration Projects* focusing on the primary prevention of type 2 diabetes in AI/AN adults with prediabetes and *CVD risk reduction* in those with type 2 diabetes were added, but only the former SDPI grantees were eligible to apply for the newer grants. The awardees included 36 *Diabetes Prevention Demonstration Project* (DPP) grantees and 30 *Healthy Heart Demonstration Project* grantees for a total of 399 SDPI grantees (i.e., competitive and community-directed). As of September 2005, the planning year for these grantees ended; the intervention will occur in Years 2-4, with Year 5 focusing on transmitting lessons learned.

In the original SPDI grants, the local community selected the focus, but with the competitive grants, all the grantees will implement the core components of the intervention (16 week modified Diabetes Prevention Program (DPP) Lifestyle Balance Curriculum – see Intervention section of this report), but aspects of their intervention may vary. The *Diabetes Prevention Demonstration Project* grantees will screen community members for diabetes risk at community events and refer high risk individuals for testing for diabetes and prediabetes. The goals for each participant include weight loss, making healthier food choices, and increased physical activity. The intervention will include education, lifestyle coaching, dietary modification, weight loss, and physical activity. A comprehensive evaluation of the competitive grantees is planned to answer questions about program effectiveness and outcomes based on solid, statistically accurate and timely data.

Healthy Children, Healthy Families and Healthy Communities Initiative. The goal of this pilot IHS Head Start program was to halt the increasing trend of obesity in young children and type 2 diabetes in youth by promoting healthy lifestyle development and change among Head Start children, families, staff, and their communities. The focus of the program was on nutrition, physical fitness, community mobilization, and environmental policy.

Beginning in January 2001, five tribal Head Start pilot sites located in rural areas developed obesity and diabetes prevention interventions in their local communities. These sites included: Eastern Band of Cherokee Head Start, North Carolina; Northern Cheyenne Head Start, Montana; Red Cliff Band of Lake Superior Chippewa Early Head Start, Wisconsin; San Felipe Pueblo Head Start, New Mexico; and Winnebago Tribe Head Start, Nebraska. (One of these sites participated for only 1 year due to lack of staff). The Head Start sites did not receive grant funding; thus, collaboration with their community partners was vital. However, the IHS Head Start Program and the IHS Division of Diabetes Treatment and Prevention provided training and technical assistance through quarterly meetings and on-site consultation visits by health experts.

For 3 years, each pilot site implemented a comprehensive multifaceted set of interventions for four target groups: Head Start children, parents/family, Head Start staff, and communities. These interventions were based on each community's needs and incorporated traditional values of AI/AN communities. Each site was required to have a key community health partner; for example, the Special Supplemental Nutrition Program for Women, Infants and Children (WIC), the CDC's Racial and Ethnic Approaches to Community Health (REACH) program or the SDPI. Interventions focused on the development of healthy habits rather than on short term quick-fix diets or rapid loss of body weight. Examples of some of the interventions include:

- The San Felipe Pueblo Head Start Program purchased and implemented a physical education and activity program for preschoolers. They also provided nutrition education to home day care providers and their Head Start site staff by a registered dietician from a partner Diabetes Prevention Program.
- The Winnebago Tribe Head Start increased the utilization of their fitness center by staff, parents and community members with incentives and strengthened bonds with their community partners by sponsoring quarterly pot lucks and organizing cross-training events in addition to other interventions.

A process evaluation of this pilot was conducted at each site (IHS, 2005a). Key findings indicated that: (1) sustainability was achieved through the continuation of many of the individual site activities in some form; (2) staff and parents gave favorable ratings to the initiative; (3) community capacity building occurred; (4) pilot sites appreciated the initial quarterly and subsequent tri-annual face-to-face meetings and resource materials provided by the IHS Head Start Program; and (5) solutions favor prevention, early intervention and lifelong strategies that promote health and are culturally sensitive. Lessons learned as a result of this pilot are being disseminated through training and technical assistance efforts, information dissemination, and presentations at regional meetings.

The primary barrier faced by all the pilot sites was high turnover of Head Start staff and community partner programs. Other barriers faced by some but not all of the sites included: high prevalence of obesity in the children, remote locations of the Head Start centers, few safe areas to walk or no sidewalks, unleashed dogs, small kitchen to prepare meals and snacks, limited outdoor space for physical activity, aging facilities inadequate for physical activities, lack of playground equipment for children, lack of participation by adult employees in physical fitness activities, and difficulty obtaining evaluation measures from the sites.

IHS Obesity Data. The Government Performance Results Act (GPRA) requires federal agencies to demonstrate that they are using their funds effectively toward meeting their missions. The law requires agencies to have a 5-year Strategic Plan in place and to submit annual Performance Plans and Reports with their budget requests. The Strategic Plan describes long term goals, and the Annual Performance Plan describes what the agency intends to accomplish toward those goals with their annual budget. Thus, the Plan contains specific performance measures for a 1-year period with long term performance goals; the Annual Performance Report then describes how the agency measured up against the performance targets set in the Performance Plan. IHS uses a Resource and Patient Management System (RPMS) clinical software application called the Clinical Reporting System (CRS) for national reporting as well as local and Area monitoring of GPRA clinical performance measures. Health care facilities can track local clinical performance continuously through CRS. Additionally, the IHS generates aggregated quarterly GPRA reports from local site or service unit data.

There is a distinction between those who are eligible for IHS services and those who use the services. The IHS service population consists of AI/ANs identified as eligible for IHS services (e.g., approximately 60 percent of all AI/ANs residing in the U.S.). The IHS user population is based on estimates from the IHS Patient Registration System and consists of those who receive direct or contract health services from IHS or tribally-operated programs.

IHS FY 04 and 05 GPRA performance measures for obesity included the following (IHS, 2005b):

- *Obesity Assessment Measure:* ***Proportion of patients for whom BMI data can be measured.*** The national average (across all IHS Areas) for body mass index (BMI) in Fiscal Year (FY) 2004 was obtained on 60 percent of active clinical patients. Reasons for a lack of adequate BMI data include lack of nursing staff and a lack of time in IHS clinics to do these measurements. Sites often had weight, but not height measurements for adults. An additional challenge is that children's height and weight measurements are not entered on the same day as required by CRS logic. The FY 2005 target was to increase the FY 2004 rate by 5 percent to 65 percent; the FY 05 national average rose to 64 percent. The goal for 2010 is 90 percent. Exhibit 4 shows the IHS Area-specific percentages of BMI assessments conducted in FY 04 and FY 05. (Note: This measure was used until FY 05, but is no longer a GPRA measure).
- *Childhood Weight Control Measure.* ***Establish the baseline rate for children ages 2-5 with a BMI of 95 percent or higher.*** The FY 2006 target is to establish the proportion of children ages 2-5 with a BMI of 95 percent or higher, and the FY 2007 target is to maintain the rate of children with a BMI of 95 percent or higher at the FY 2006 level.

IHS BMI data on 60 percent of all AI/AN active users age 2-74 (e.g., N=463,392) indicates that the percentage of AI/ANs who are either overweight or obese increased between FY 2000 –FY 2004 from 67 percent to 70 percent; however, this percentage is similar to rate for U.S adults who were obese or overweight in 2000 – 65 percent. The percentage of AI/ANs who are obese increased from 41 percent in FY 2000 to 44 percent in FY 2004; this is higher than the percentage of U.S adults who were obese in 2000 – 31 percent. See Exhibit 5.

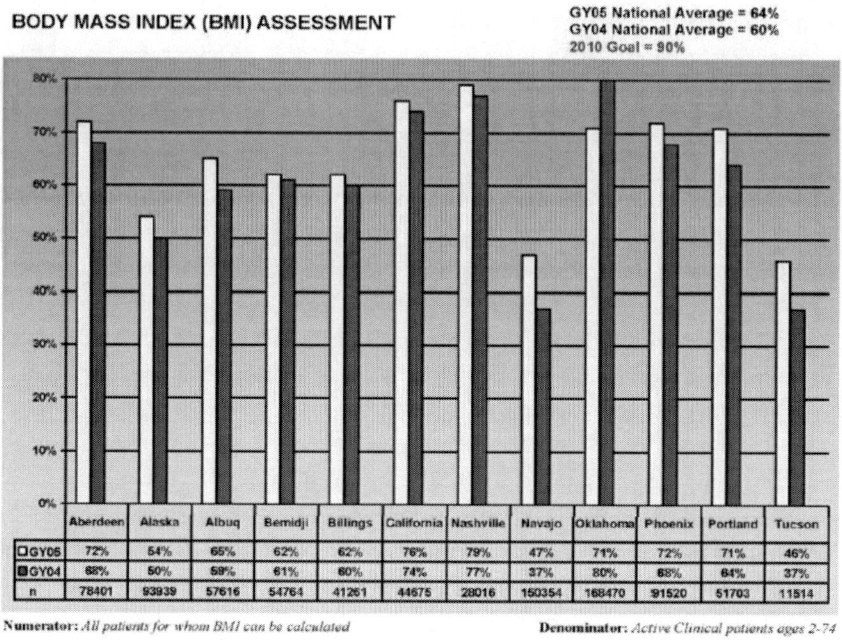

	Aberdeen	Alaska	Albuq	Bemidji	Billings	California	Nashville	Navajo	Oklahoma	Phoenix	Portland	Tucson
GY05	72%	54%	65%	62%	62%	76%	79%	47%	71%	72%	71%	46%
GY04	68%	50%	59%	61%	60%	74%	77%	37%	80%	68%	64%	37%
n	78401	93939	57616	54764	41261	44675	28016	150354	168470	91520	51703	11514

Exhibit 4.

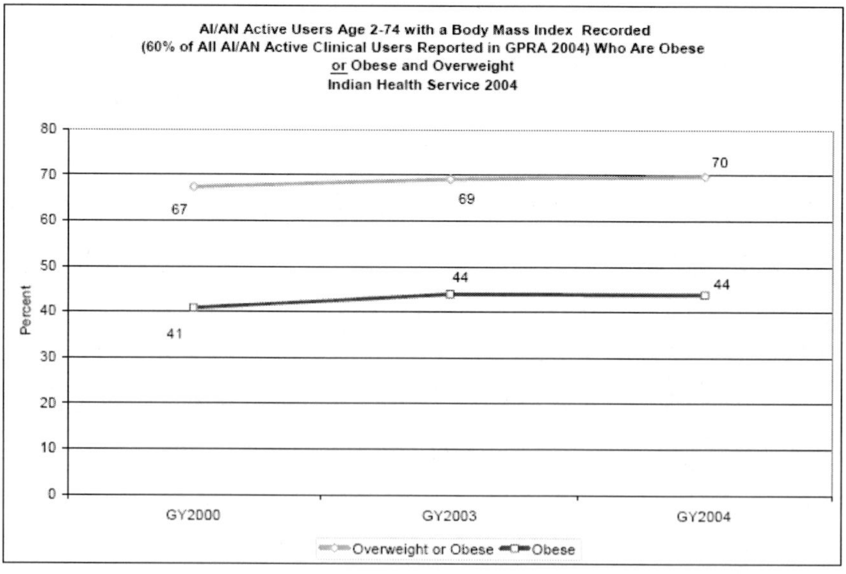

Exhibit 5.

The same IHS data also indicates that there are important differences in BMI by the 12 IHS Areas (Cullen, 2005). See Table 5. IHS staff asked that these Areas not be identified. In FY 2004, for overweight and obesity combined (N=322,952), there is a range from 62.1 percent in Area A to 77.5 percent in Area L and for obesity alone (N=203,370), the range is from 34.6 percent in Area A to 57.8 percent in Area L.

A physician key informant identified community normalization and resignation as barriers to obesity prevention. This physician indicated that a tipping point may be reached when 50% or more of the population are overweight/obese in terms of the community being resigned to the issue. Additionally, in the past, doctors themselves may not have known how to approach the obesity problem.

Currently, IHS is working on an important project that will examine their RPMS clinical data from 1999-present pertaining to height and weight for the 0-2 and 2-6 age groups from all 12 IHS areas. The focus of this study is to assess trends over time and answer questions about when obesity/overweight begins in AI/ANs. Does it begin from birth – 2 years, or does it begin in the 2-6 age range or are both age ranges involved in the origins of problem? Knowing the answer to these questions will be very helpful to IHS and others in terms of the most appropriate time to intervene. The IHS clinical sample has several biases; for example, 1) it includes only those persons who come to an IHS clinic for a well child visit or a health-related reason; 2) tribes that compact their health services submit their data on a voluntary basis only; and 3) overweight/obese children may be more likely to get their height and weight measured.

However findings from this clinical sample could be compared to a school-based sample in order to examine the extent to which these biases influence the findings (Kileen, Martin, 2006).

Some tribes are implementing obesity prevention programs. For example, one IHS site that has documented reductions in the percentage of toddlers and youth who are overweight or obese attributes this to the motivation of the community to be healthier and having several full time registered dietitians. Health messages at this site have not been focused on obesity, but rather being active and eating healthy. In fact, their flyer states: "You benefit from being active whether or not you lose weight." Community members at this site are involved in nutrition education at elementary schools, breastfeeding promotion and walking programs for youth and adults. Additionally, staff is encouraged to measure height and weight of infants and children.

Table 5. Percentage of Obese and Obese Combined with Overweight by IHS Areas in FY 2004*

	# Obese	% Obese	# Overweight or Obese	# PTs with BMI	Area % Obese & Overweight
Area A	16256	34.6%	29215	47017	62.1%
Area B	22091	40.1%	37466	55039	68.0%
Area C	34106	42.2%	54639	80769	67.6%
Area D	10324	42.2%	16796	24439	68.7%
Area E	15074	43.6%	24268	34549	70.2%
Area F	23159	44.5%	36904	52018	70.9%
Area G	13723	46.1%	21353	29758	71.8%
Area H	12453	46.3%	19373	26911	72.0%
Area I	15347	47.0%	23335	32652	71.5%
Area J	9801	48.8%	14753	20085	73.5%
Area K	28408	51.5%	41332	55622	74.3%
Area L	2618	57.8%	3511	4533	77.5%
N=	203370		322925	463392	

* Percent of obese and overweight are calculated from active clinical patients with BMI assessments only.

On the T.R.A.I.L. (Together Raising Awareness for Indian Life) to Diabetes Prevention. This project involves a recreation, nutrition, and diabetes prevention program that takes place at Boys & Girls Clubs located in 40 Native American communities. It is supported by a collaborative partnership between the National Congress of American Indians, IHS, Boys & Girls Clubs of America, Nike, and FirstPic, Inc., and is currently in Year 4. IHS contributes funding annually to support one full-time equivalent program coordinator, supplies and training for each of the sites. New T.R.A.I.L. sites also receive NikeGO product grants of $10,000 in the form equipment and incentives. Additionally, sites receive ongoing training and technical assistance twice a year.

A T.R.A.I.L. grant is awarded for 1 year. Each T.R.A.I.L. session runs for 3 months, so during 1 year, a site conducts two cycles of the T.R.A.I.L. curriculum with 25 children involved in each cycle. Sites are required to have a Memorandum of Understanding with their local IHS clinic or health organization and also partner with a local Head Start or early education program.

Utilizing tribal traditions, T.R.A.I.L. implements self-esteem and prevention activities to teach about nutrition, food choices and their impact on diabetes. The target age is 8-10 year olds and 50-70 percent of these children are obese. T.R.A.I.L. has four basic themes: 1) About Me and My Health, 2) Diabetes and Nutrition, 3) Making Smart Food Choices, and 4) Sharing Knowledge with Others. The curriculum includes activities outside the site (physical activity and behavioral change) as well as family orientation and community events.

An ongoing evaluation is being conducted, and its focus is on measurement of two dimensions: knowledge about diabetes, nutrition and food choices (using a pre- and post-test) and physical activity (each site has 40-60 minutes of physical activity daily). Although height and weight measures are obtained in the beginning of the program, they are not measured at the end. The evaluation will not be able to address research questions until the fourth year of the program.

The strengths of this program thus far are: (1) the interest and dedication of the communities evidenced by the creativity and local adaptations implemented at the sites; 2) popularity of the program with the target audience; and (3) use of a standardized intervention along with technical assistance and training. Evaluators indicated that challenges include: (1) lack of funding for an outside evaluator or data coordinator; (2) unfamiliarity of program staff with research methods and procedures; (3) high staff turnover at the sites; (4) difficulty getting data reports submitted; and (5) poor results in obtaining self-report data from children on activities taking place outside the Boys & Girls Clubs; for example, watching television or physical activity. Evaluators believe that the lessons learned from this evaluation will serve to strengthen the design of future evaluations.

BodyWorks. The IHS, Division of Diabetes Treatment and Prevention is collaborating with the Office of Women's Health (OWH/DHHS) to adapt the Bodyworks toolkit developed by OWH to prevent overweight and obesity in adolescent girls into a similar toolkit for AI/AN mothers and girls. After a series of focus groups conducted around the country, OWH developed a generic toolkit and tested it with consumer groups, including an AI parent group. The AI/AN kit will include the following:

- Booklet for parents outlining group sessions and a smaller booklet for adolescent girls ages 9-13 years containing games and interactive materials;

- Book of recipes obtained from registered dietitians and public health nutritionists who work with AI/AN communities as well as the National Institute of Diabetes and Digestive and Kidney Diseases (NIDDK) and the National Heart Lung and Blood Institute (NHLBI), including recipes for Native American foods and quiz and recipe cards;
- Group discussion guide;
- Food and activity journal for the adolescent girls;
- Menu-planning refrigerator magnet;
- Environmental checklist for families to evaluate home, school and community to support healthy weight;
- Two pedometers; and
- DVD (20 minutes).

BodyWorks is written at a low literacy level (i.e., 5-6th grade) for the AI/AN-adapted kit. The program involves ten 1 hour group sessions with the mothers or caregivers of the adolescent girls; two of these sessions include the girls. Parents must agree to attend the ten sessions and sign a contract. The generic toolkits will be distributed nationally using a community-based "Train-the-Trainer" model. The cost of the project was approximately $750,000 and $350,000 respectively for the generic and AI/AN adapted kits.

The consumer group of AI mothers made the following recommendations for tailoring the kit to an AI/AN audience:

- Include photos and other designs that reflect the culture of AI/ANs. Include also foods and recipes that reflect AI/AN cooking and meals;
- Include symbols of the AI/AN culture such as animals or drums and consider other traditions such as storytelling or crafts as elements to be incorporated into the design;
- Consider using a contemporary interpretation of traditional symbols, and avoid using the motifs of any specific tribe;
- Research food choices, cooking styles and physical activities of typical AN girls and incorporate this information;
- Identify AI video producers who could adapt a script for the AI/AN audience. Key messages for the video should be: (1) cooking healthy meals can be quick and inexpensive; (2) eating together helps families communicate and encourages healthy food choices; (3) shopping for healthy foods helps to plan nutritious meals; (4) limiting sedentary pastimes can offer time for physical activity;

and (5) there are many types of physical activity that are healthy and fun; and

- Determine the best way to disseminate the kit to an AI/AN audience.

The AI/AN version uses a similar format and structure as the generic version, although it has been tailored for an AI/AN audience through incorporation of the comments from the AI mother focus group and IHS staff who work with AI/AN community members and who may also be Native American themselves. Dissemination of the AI/AN version is planned for sometime in FY 2007, and a "Train-the-Trainer" model will be used. Distribution will be across the Indian health diabetes network that includes the Area diabetes consultants, the model diabetes programs, and the SDPI grantees. IHS will also involve the Area health promotion/disease prevention consultants, public health nursing, behavioral health specialists, physical fitness trainers and specialists, registered dietitians, tribal and Bureau of Indian Affairs school staff, and health educators in the dissemination.

An evaluation of the generic version will begin in fall 2006. The evaluation of the AI/AN toolkit will include process measures related to the implementation and distribution of BodyWorks and outcome measures such as participants' experiences with implementing and achieving success in increasing physical activity and practicing healthier eating habits. Participant's pre- and post-test scores on knowledge, attitudes and behaviors around nutrition and physical activity may be collected. Qualitiative data may also be collected from local trainers and volunteer participants through key informant interviews. Preliminary results for the AI/AN version may be available at the end of FY 2008 or mid-FY 2009.

Tailoring Dietary Guidelines. IHS is working on a project that will involve tailoring the U.S Dietary Guidelines for AI/ANs. This effort planned to begin in Fall, 2006 will take into account the spiritual, social and health values of indigenous foods; Native culture and traditions; the environment; behavioral, mental and physical issues; and spiritual aspects of Native life. The tailored guidelines will be simplified and written using a lower literacy level than the national dietary guidelines and will focus on foods versus nutrients. The project will be implemented by a contractor and will include guidance from an advisory group.

Key Informants from IHS

Kelly Acton, MD., Division of Diabetes Treatment and Prevention, Albuquerque NM, IHS.

Brenda Boussard, Consultant for the Healthy Children, Healthy Families and Healthy Communities Initiative

Eric Broderick, Office of the Administrator, SAMHSA, Washington D.C.

Tammy Brown, Division of Diabetes Treatment and Prevention, Albuquerque, NM, IHS. Jean Charles-Azure, Headquarters, Rockville MD, IHS.

Terry Cullen, MD, Headquarters, Rockville, MD, IHS. Jennifer Daniel, National Programs Albuquerque, NM, IHS. Honahnie, Dealva, IHS, Phoenix, AZ

Candace Jones, National Programs Albuquerque, NM, IHS. Martin Kileen, National Programs Albuquerque, NM, IHS.

Zeenat Mahal, Epdemiology Center, Inter Tribal Council of Arizona, Phoenix AZ Kelly Moore, Division of Diabetes Treatment and Prevention, NM, IHS.

Jonelle Rowe, Office on Woman's Health, DHHS, Washington D.C. Amy Staubs, FirstPic, Incorporated, Crofton, MD

Cheryl Wilson, National Programs Albuquerque, NM, IHS.

National Institutes of Health (NIH)

The following NIH activities will be described in this section:

- NIH Obesity Research;
- The Diabetes Prevention Program, National Institute of Diabetes and Digestive and Kidney Diseases (NIDDK);
- Sharing Wisdom Study (NIDDK);
- Diabetes Education in Tribal Schools Program (NIDDK);
- National Diabetes Education Program;
- Bright Start Program, National Heart, Lung and Blood Institute (NHLBI);
- Community-Responsive Interventions to Reduce Cardiovascular Risk in AI/ANs (NHLBI);
- Primordial Toddler Overweight and Tooth Decay Study (NHLBI);
- Obesity and Cardiac Risk in American Indian Children (NHLBI); and
- Honoring the Gift of Heart Health (NHLBI);

NIH Obesity Research

The NIH supports a broad spectrum of obesity-related research, including molecular, genetic, behavioral, environmental, clinical, and epidemiologic studies. An NIH Obesity Research Task Force was established in April 2003 and is co-chaired by the Director of the National Institute of Diabetes and Digestive and Kidney Diseases (NIDDK) and the National Heart, Lung, and Blood Institute (NHLBI). This group meets quarterly. The Task Force was responsible for developing a *Strategic Plan for NIH Obesity Research* (NIH, 2004).

The purpose of the *Strategic Plan for NIH Obesity Research* is to provide a guide for coordinating obesity research activities across the NIH and for enhancing the development of new research efforts. The goals of the Plan are organized under four themes:

- Research toward preventing and treating obesity through lifestyle modification;
- Research toward preventing and treating obesity through pharmacological, surgical or other medical approaches;
- Research toward breaking the link between obesity and its associated health conditions; and
- Crosscutting research topics, including health disparities, technology, fostering of multidisciplinary and interdisciplinary research teams, investigator training, translational research, and education/outreach efforts.

Extramurally, the NIH supports both investigator-initiated research projects and research that results from NIH-initiated efforts – solicitations for grant applications and contract proposals. The NIH also supports an Intramural Research Program pertaining to obesity research. NIH obesity funding based on actual grants, contracts, research, and other mechanisms of support for FY 2003 was $379 million; for FY 2004, 422 million; for FY and 2005, 519 million. Estimates of this funding for FY 2006 and FY 2007 are for $519 million.

The Computer Retrieval of Information on Scientific Projects (CRISP) is a biomedical database system that includes information on research projects (mostly extramural) that are supported by DHHS. The website for this system is located at: http://crisp.cit.nih.gov. Queries of CRISP for 2006 revealed 12 projects pertaining to obesity and AIs and 67 similar projects for the years between 2000-2006. Examples of 2006 projects relevant to obesity and AIs include:

- *Walking to Health for American Indian Children.* This pilot intervention involves a school-based policy change to incorporate a daily 1-mile walk for third and fourth grade students as part of the school day in three elementary schools on two Indian reservations in northern Minnesota. The outcomes that will be examined include: change in BMI, change in body composition, change in average daily physical activity, and change in attitudes and preferences for physical activity. Funded by NIDDK, this project began in September 2004 and will end in May 2006.
- *Early Socioeconomic and Psychological Risk for Obesity.* This research will use ongoing U.S. and international longitudinal studies to explore the behavioral and psychological factors that cause additive risk for obesity in populations at risk. The study samples include AI preschool children, Costa Rican children, Chilean children, and Finnish adults. The hypothesis is that children are put at risk for obesity by biologic and social factors including poverty, parental mental health, and parental-decision making about childhood nutrition and activity. This project began in June 2001 and will end in May 2006.

National Institute of Diabetes and Digestive and Kidney Diseases (NIDDK)

The Diabetes Prevention Program (DPP). The purpose, methodology and results of this study are fully described in the Intervention section of this report.

Diabetes Prevention Program Outcomes Study (DPPOS). Eighty-five percent of the initial DPP cohort (including AI/ANs as well as other groups) is enrolled in the DPPOS that began in 2003 and will end in January 2009. At the end of the DPP, all its participants received the 16 week lifestyle intervention. The original three DPP intervention groups are now receiving the following types of interventions in this study:

- DPP placebo group is receiving a *modified* lifestyle intervention through regular group meetings;

- DPP metformin group is receiving the drug metformin and the *modified* lifestyle group intervention through regular groups meetings; and
- DPP intensive life style intervention group is receiving *intensive* lifestyle group intervention through regular, but a reduced number of group meetings.

The DPPOS is examining the long-term effect of diet and exercise and metformin, on the delay of type 2 diabetes in participants of the DPP. Key research issues include: 1) the maintenance of weight loss; 2) the occurrence of diabetes; 2) the occurrence of cardiovascular disease and risk factors for CVD, atherosclerosis, and microvascular disease; and 3) examination of these topics in men versus women and in minority populations.

Four of the 26 DPPOS clinical centers sample only tribal members (e.g., Salt River, Zuni, Gila River, and Shiprock). One data coordinating center exists and is funded by NIDDK. NIDDK, CDC and IHS are co-funders of this study with the NIDDK contributing approximately $9 million per year.

This study is the longest running weight loss study conducted to date. Preliminary results in terms of weight maintenance and loss are promising. Findings pertaining to CVD and diabetes are blinded and will not be available until the fifth or sixth years of the study. Furthermore, it will take several years after the study ends to analyze all of the data that is being collected.

There are several important lessons that have been learned to date. First, researchers have learned effective ways of enrolling participants. The AI individuals who participated in the DPP continue to participate in this study and have shown a high interest and commitment in these clinical trials. These are persons who do not have a disease, but rather are at risk for diabetes. AIs involved in this study are motivated due to their family histories of diabetes and concern for their children. Another important lesson is that different agencies can work very well together. A Steering Committee for this project meets three times a year and has been involved in both the DPP and the DPPOS. Members of these agencies are also involved in writing groups focused on study findings.

Sharing Wisdom Study. In 2001, NIDDK funded the University of New Mexico's Native American Diabetes Program (NADP) to conduct a 5-year randomized controlled trial to develop and test the effectiveness of a healthy lifestyle educational intervention focusing on reducing risk factors for type 2 diabetes. The target population for this study was non-diabetic urban-dwelling

AI women (Albuquerque, New Mexico) aged 18-40 years. The study was funded for $300,000 per year and ends in December 2006 (Herman, 2006).

Participants were recruited from the urban community at large through flyers, word-of-mouth and local media messages. At baseline, 73 percent of the 200 women were overweight or obese, 21 percent had pre-diabetes, and 28 percent met criteria for metabolic syndrome. Nearly three- fourths of the women reported a family history of type 2 diabetes. Two hundred participants were randomized into two equal groups, an intervention group and a comparison group that received a delayed intervention after all their clinical measures were completed. Clinical measures were obtained at baseline, 6-months (immediately post intervention), 12-months and 18-months. The 12 and 18 month results were not available for inclusion in this report.

A culturally tailored healthy lifestyle curriculum (based on the earlier *Strong in Body and Spirit* curriculum[1]) was used after obtaining feedback from focus groups. Pilot testing revealed that it is important not to assume that all Native Americans practice their traditions to the same degree or that they share similar traditions. The intervention consisted of five sessions (2 hours each) held monthly for 5 months and led by community-based Native American health educators. These sessions addressed the topics of physical activity, eating more vegetables and less fat, reducing intake of sweetened beverages and processed high sugar foods, social support, and maintenance of healthy lifestyle behavior changes. The sessions included a few minutes of moderate or light physical activity, discussions of behavior changes over the past month, didactic lessons and discussion, and healthy behavior goal setting for the month ahead.

Participants were contacted frequently by mail, phone and email and had an in-person contact at least every 6 months. They were also given a payment of $50 for each clinic visit and reimbursement of child care and transportation costs for clinic visits and classes as needed. There was no cash payment for attendance at intervention group sessions. Of the 200 eligible women participants at baseline, 82 percent completed 6 month clinic measures, while 77 percent completed the 12-month measures.

Although these women had a strong interest in diabetes prevention, and many were motivated by a family history of diabetes and a desire to share prevention strategies with family members, retention was a challenge. The women had multiple roles including childcare, work and school. Although sessions were held on evenings and weekends, they found it difficult to attend. Their schedules changed as their schooling and part-time work schedules shifted. They frequently moved within local areas or out-of-the area, and their cell phone numbers changed frequently. Over half (53 percent) of the 100 women assigned to the intervention group attended three or more of the five intervention group sessions. Only 18 percent of these participants attended all 5 classes; 17 percent attended 4 classes, 18 percent attended 3 classes, 14 percent attended 2 classes, 13 percent attended 1 class and 20 percent attended 0 classes.

Preliminary changes at 6 months compared to baseline show significant changes in the intervention group as compared to the control group for self-reported dietary patterns (e.g., increased vegetable consumption, decreased fats and sweets intake) and decreased diastolic blood pressure, body composition, and self-reported physical activity. Exit interviews revealed an appreciation for class discussions and the group problem solving that took place during these sessions. Among overweight women, more intervention than control women lost weight (59.7 percent versus 39.3 percent). Seventy-four percent of the intervention group met physical activity recommendations of at least 150 minutes/week of moderate intensity activity or 60 minutes/week of vigorous activity compared to 64 percent at baseline, while in the control group the percentage of women meeting activity recommendations declined. These 6-month findings indicate that a less intensive lifestyle intervention for young at-risk women can reduce risks for type 2 diabetes (Allen et al., 2006a; Allen et al., 2006b).

Intervention participants significantly increased their stage of change (e.g., pre-contemplation, contemplation, preparation, action, maintenance) as compared to the control group women for eating at least three servings of vegetables and choosing healthier snacks. However, state of change for exercise did not significantly change for either group.

The control group women made some healthy life style changes on their own, perhaps due to the clinical measures that were periodically recorded. Both groups had significantly reduced waist circumference, total caloric intake, total cholesterol and LDL cholesterol, and hours/day spent watching TV.

Focus groups were held with a select sample of the participants to obtain suggestions for improving future interventions. The following are lessons learned that will be implemented in the next study:

- Interventions must be responsive to the differing social realities of urban AI women (Willging et al., 2006). These young women wanted a less traditional approach than those living on reservations; for example, a less family-oriented and culture specific approach;

- Classroom education about physical activity and social support for activity proved insufficient to stimulate increases in fitness levels. Thus, in the next study, participants will be provided with a membership in a private exercise facility and incentives for joining this organization. They will be able to participate at convenient times according to their changing schedules;
- The intervention should be designed so that urban women can participate individually or with their best friends or buddies at varying times. Thus, in the next study, they will acquire their exercise and nutrition information on the Internet. However, because women still wanted the option to attend face-to-face sessions, these will be conducted as voluntary sessions;
- The upper age limit of study participants will be increased to 49 instead of 40 in order to decrease the dropout rate due to pregnancy and increase interventions with women at higher risk for type 2 diabetes due to increasing age; and
- Highly trained Native American staff will continue to contact and guide participants when clinical measures are recorded and throughout the intervention.

Diabetes Education in Tribal Schools (DETS) Program. The DETS Project is partnering with Tribal Colleges and Universities (TCUs) to develop a K-12 diabetes-science prevention curriculum for tribal and other schools serving AI/AN students. The curriculum teaches the science of diabetes within a cultural context and builds individual, family and community knowledge. Obesity prevention information on healthy lifestyle choices for children and families at risk (e.g. nutrition and physical activity) is included. This project is also designed to encourage tribal students to prepare for biomedical careers. Tribal colleges were the only entities that could apply for these grants, and eight were selected.

This project began in 2001 and evolved as a result of meetings between the Federal Interagency Diabetes Mellitus Coordinating Committee (DMICC) and the Tribal Leader's Diabetes Committee/IHS. The lead agency is NIDDK and collaborating partners and co-funders include CDC and IHS. In FY 2001, funding was available for up to five planning grant awards made to Tribal Colleges and Universities (TCUs). In FY 2002, grants were awarded to eight TCUs. These awards will continue for additional years.

The curriculum has been developed in three grade areas, K-4; 5-8, and 9-12 respectively. The DETS curriculum lessons are currently being piloted and beta tested at tribal and tribal member schools in proximity to the 8 TCUs on the DETS team. A number of additional schools, "sister sites," have been added to include diverse regions in the U.S. not represented by the 8 TCUs. The completed curriculum will be available at the end of 2008, and the plan is to disseminate it to schools that have significant AI enrollment. Tribal (K-12) schools throughout the country have been identified to allow for broad evaluation of the curricula and to provide satellite sites for marketing and dissemination. The DETS K-4 curriculum incorporates the *Eagle Book Series*, four vividly illustrated children's books developed by the Native Diabetes Wellness Program, CDC, and IHS's Division of Diabetes Treatment and Prevention. These books feature a colorful cast of wise animal characters who share with children the wisdom of healthy eating, physical activity and learning from their elders about living in balance. The books are popular with American Indian/Alaska Native children throughout the U.S. and Canada.

Three agencies (i.e., NIDDK, CDC and IHS) are involved in the evaluation that is built into the project. The project has an external advisory committee consisting of curriculum experts, AI groups, and tribal leadership. There are several evaluation teams. One of these teams focuses on evaluation of the curricula specifically. The teachers are to complete instruments during pilot, beta and field-testing and also will conduct pre and posttesting of the students. In order to examine how the curriculum is received, the second evaluation team is conducting ethnographic interviews with five sets of persons (teachers, parents, community advisory groups, informal community leaders, and TCU personnel) at each TCU. Approximately 90 persons will be interviewed. A third team, the scientific review committee, examines the curricula for scientific accuracy and consistency. The TCU curriculum committees provide oversight for cultural relevance and historical accuracy. NIDDK is utilizing an external education group that specializes in curriculum development to review the entire curricula, with input from the TCU subcommittees, for educational presentation and consistency across the three educational groupings.

National Diabetes Education Program (NDEP). This program was founded in 1997 and is a federally sponsored initiative that involves public and private partners to improve treatment and outcomes for people with diabetes, promote early diagnosis and prevent the onset of diabetes. NIDDK and the Division of Diabetes Translation of the CDC jointly sponsor NDEP, with the participation of over 200 partner agencies. The target audiences of the NDEP include: people with or at risk for type 2 diabetes, with special attention to minority groups including AIs and ANs; older adults; health care providers payers; purchasers; and policy makers.

There are five principle objectives of the NDEP:

- Increase awareness of the seriousness of diabetes, its risk factors, and strategies for preventing diabetes and its complications among high risk groups;
- Improve understanding about diabetes and its control and promote better self- management behaviors among people with diabetes;
- Improve health care providers' understanding of diabetes and its control and promote an integrated approach to care;
- Promote health care policies that improve the quality of and access to diabetes care; and
- Reduce disparities in health and racial and ethnic populations disproportionately affected by diabetes.

There are three primary NDEP public education campaigns: 1) *Control Your Diabetes For Life,* 2) Be Smart About Your Heart. Control the ABCs of Diabetes, and 3) Small Steps. Big Rewards. Prevent type 2 Diabetes (i.e., Small Steps). Because the Small Steps Campaign is the most relevant for obesity prevention, only it will be discussed here. Based on the science of the DPP (DPP Research Group, 2002), Small Steps was launched in February 2003 and is targeted to health care providers and adults who are over 45 years of age and overweight. The primary components of the campaign include: public service advertising (e.g., radio, TV, print ads), publicity campaigns involving events in cities across the country, a health care provider's "GAME PLAN" toolkit, consumer "GAME PLAN" materials, and a Speaker's Kit.

NDEP achievements between 1997-2003 include reaching 1 billion persons through print and broadcast media and disseminating 2 million consumer publications along with 350,000 publications to health care providers. Broadcast Public Service Announcements (PSAs) were valued at $30.3 million and print PSAs reached 53.4 million in circulation (NDEP).

In 2004, the NDEP released a tailored version of the *Small Steps* materials to at-risk communities including AI/ANs. Messages in the campaign stress that while huge changes are often unrealistic, moderate changes in lifestyle – such as taking a 30-minute walk every day – can cut dramatically a person's risk for diabetes. The tag line for the AI/AN tailored campaign is: *We have the Power to Prevent Diabetes.* One of the lessons learned has been that the AI/ANs need to be involved in these campaigns from the beginning so that they have ownership of the campaign, the right messages are disseminated, and materials are disseminated to those who need to see them. *We have the Power* was piloted, but there has not been an ongoing evaluation of outcomes.

NDEP includes several other activities pertaining to AI/ANs and obesity prevention. The NDEP AI/AN Work Group includes AI/AN health professionals and community leaders who advise the NDEP on the development of public health messages and on the dissemination of campaign materials to Indian health programs, tribes and communities. Members work with a contractor in the development, testing and evaluation of the health messages. The current emphasis of the group is on using cost-effective methods to make materials available to a wide audience. The Work Group is involved in monthly conference calls and meets in-person on a yearly basis

The Association of American Indian Physicians (AAIP) is also a component of the NDEP. This group is charged with developing and disseminating culturally tailored messages for AI/AN communities, and they work in partnership with the NDEP AI/AN Work Group. They are also responsible for building the capacity of national and regional organizations to promote community-based interventions and improving the capacity of local health care providers to provide appropriate information. In 1997, the AAPI conducted a series of focus groups to gather input from tribal leaders, Indian health professionals, and AI community members to guide the development of culturally appropriate diabetes education materials for NDEP (Roubideaux et al., 2000). Participants in these groups preferred materials adapted to the specific culture, language and traditions of the local tribe or community, if feasible. They also wanted more educational materials available in their communities and schools and requested more materials with information on diet and exercise. CDC funds the work of the AAIP through a cooperative agreement.

Some of the key activities that the Workgroup and Physicians Group have collaborated on are:

- *Move-It! And Reduce Your Risk of Diabetes program.* Campaign packets for AI/AN youth ages 12-18 were developed. These packets include several posters depicting Native American youth involved in physical activities, a print advertisement designed to be included in a newsletter, a fact sheet with information about diabetes type 2, a resource guide, and a list of suggested activities and ways to use the materials. In 2004, OMH provided funding to 10 schools serving AI/AN youth so they could develop activities that use *Move It!*

materials, and AAIP selected four schools to serve as models for other *Move It!* programs.

In August 2002, the “Move-It” Campaign materials were mailed to all Bureau of Indian Affairs schools in the U.S. CDC funded an evaluation to determine the recall and utilization of the packet and to gather in-depth input on the materials from staff in the BIA schools (ORC, Macro 2003). Of the 181 schools that participated in telephone calls, 52.5 percent recalled receiving the packet. One-third of those who received the packet used the materials themselves, and two-thirds passed them onto someone else. Among those who recalled receiving the materials, the most frequent uses of the information were displaying the posters in the school, using the fact sheet to teach about diabetes, and using the materials with an existing activity.

Key recommendations included: (1) sending materials early in the school year so that they could be incorporated into lesson plans; (2) providing “how to” steps for addressing barriers that discourage utilization of the materials; and (3) changing the focus from increased awareness to increased behavior change. IHS and AAIP plan to disseminate the packets broadly to IHS Diabetes Prevention programs and to BIA schools for the second wave of the campaign.

- *The NDEP AI/AN Community Partnerships Guide: Supplement and Activity Plans* was developed by the AI/AN Workgroup and the AAIP to encourage community-based activities that provide education about diabetes prevention and treatment and it includes specific examples of such activities (CDC, 2004).

NIDDK’s Phoenix Epidemiology and Clinical Research Branch. For a discussion of the AI- related research conducted by this group, refer to the Gila River Indian Community Section of this report, NIDDK Research Presentations.

The National Heart, Lung, and Blood Institute (NHLBI)

Bright Start Program. Awarded to a grantee at the University of Minnesota in January 2005 for 4 years, this study targets kindergarten and first grade AI children on the Pine Ridge and Rosebud reservations (North and South Dakota). The study will develop and test the efficacy of a school environmental intervention, augmented with a family household environmental intervention, to reduce excessive weight gain by increasing physical activity and health dietary practices. The three primary goals of the intervention are to: increase physical activity at school to 60 minutes/day; modify school meals and snacks and classroom food practices; and involve families in making behavioral and environmental changes at home.

A group randomized controlled trial with 14 schools randomized to two conditions (intervention and control) for 16 months will be used. Two cohorts of kindergarten children will be followed through the end of first grade. The primary child outcome measures are BMI and percent body fat. Secondary measures include child's total daily physical activity, nutrient analysis of school meals and snacks, and assessment of classroom food and physical activity practices. Child measures will occur at the beginning (baseline) and end of kindergarten and at the end of first grade. Parent assessment will include measures of household food availability and parent reports of their own and child eating and physical activity behaviors. Parents will be surveyed at baseline and the end of first grade.

Community-Responsive Interventions to Reduce Cardiovascular Risk in AI/ANs. NHLBI has invited applications for cooperative agreements to conduct 5-year studies in AI/AN communities to test the effectiveness of behavioral interventions to promote the adoption of healthy lifestyles and/or improve behaviors related to cardiovascular risk in AI/AN adults and/or children at high risk for cardiovascular disease (e.g., weight reduction, regular physical activity, and smoking cessation). This initiative focuses on primary prevention and its emphasis is on developing and testing culturally appropriate interventions that could be incorporated into community health care systems or public health approaches in Native communities. Approximately $8.8 million is available from the NHLBI over 5 years, and it is anticipated that up to three awards will be made from this Request for Proposals (RFP). The start date is September 1, 2006.

The target population is AI/AN adults or children at high risk for CVD, but free of clinical CVD. CVD risk factors used to identify eligible participants may be either behavior or biological and could include obesity and sedentary lifestyle. Behavioral or environmental approaches to behavioral changes may be utilized (e.g., increasing the availability of fresh fruits and vegetables). The research design must be experimental with either an individual or family randomized design or a quasi-experimental design with community or school randomization, and it must include an intensive intervention group and a comparison group. Interventions can be up to 2 years in duration and targeted behaviors include increasing regular physical activity, reducing or preventing overweight and obesity, and improving diet. Outcome measures include BMI or body weight for diet and physical activity, pedometer measures for physical activity, nutrient biomarkers as measures of dietary intake, and other measures.

The RFP specifies that the research plan be consistent with community attitudes and readiness for change; for example, strategies may involve using traditional AI/AN games, sports and dances to increase physical activity or re-introducing traditional AI/AN diets which are low in saturated fat. The intervention program should also be designed so that it can be sustained within the entire community.

Primordial Toddler Overweight and Tooth Decay Study (PTOTS). This is a 5 year overweight/obesity prevention project targeting AI children 0-3 years of age. The objectives are to test whether community and family-based interventions can alter feeding practices (e.g., breastfeeding, sugared beverage consumption, timing and type of introduction of solids) and parenting to reduce sedentary lifestyles (e.g., delayed introduction of television and creating play opportunities) in Northwest AI communities. Six tribes are partnering with the Northwest Portland Area Indian Health Board and the Kaiser Permanente Center for Health Research to implement PTOTS. The project began in September 2005.

Two tribes serve as controls, another two receive a community-only intervention, and a third set of two tribes receive both the community intervention plus a family intervention. Community interventions include: 1) raising public awareness regarding the contribution of overweight and obesity to later health conditions; 2) delivery of health education to improve the lifestyles of children; 3) changing individual family health behaviors to favor prevention of overweight in children; 4) improving public health practice in community health institutions that service children and their families; and 5) changing the environment to facilitate healthful behaviors. Each tribe will design its own interventions. Family interventions will target behavior change within families. Trained community health advocates will deliver family interventions through counseling targeting lifestyle practices. The outcomes of that this project is focusing on are early childhood overweight and early childhood caries (ECC).

In addition, the qualitative impact of the PTOTS intervention on: (1) public awareness of the overweight/dental caries link to adult health, (2) environmental changes, (3) public health practice in the Special Supplemental Nutrition Program for Women, Infants and Children (WIC) and Maternal and

Child Health (MCH) clinics and (4) behavior change among tribal members will be examined through community observations and mappings, interviews with key informants and focus groups.

Obesity and Cardiac Risk in American Indian Children. NLHBI has given a career development award to a researcher at the University of Wisconsin at Madison. The researcher's study hypothesis is that the high prevalence of obesity AI children begins in early childhood, and thus prevention efforts must be targeted at this time. The study involves a three-phase collaborative participatory research project with two Wisconsin tribal communities. The project will assess obesity prevalence and cardiac risk factors in AI children ages 0-7 years, conduct growth modeling of the familial and environmental determinants of obesity, and work in partnership with the communities to design and test community-based early intervention strategies to prevent childhood obesity and its sequelae: CVD and diabetes. This project began in September 2002 and will end in July 2006. NLHBI funding is $25,000/year.

Honoring the Gift of Heart Health. The NHLBI has developed an exciting partnership with the Indian Health Service (IHS) to focus expertise and resources on the prevention of CVD in AI/AN communities. The NHLBI Honoring the Gift of Heart Health project is a comprehensive health promotion and outreach program seeking to increase heart health awareness, knowledge, and skill among AI/ANs using a lay health worker approach. The primary purpose of the project is to provide science-based cardiovascular health (CVH) tools and training for tribal communities and consistent "standard" CVH information to AI/AN lay audiences.

The Honoring the Gift of Heart Health project focuses on educating tribal communities and tribal health care workers on cardiovascular prevention, and has begun to play a role in helping tribal communities to integrate and coordinate their CVD prevention efforts, by bringing heart health education and tailored outreach and skills training to communities and clinics throughout Indian Country.

The first phase of the project focused on the creation of culturally competent education materials to support CVD prevention efforts at the community level. These materials include the following:

- *Your Heart, Your Drum Video* – The 10-minute motivational video focuses on the issue of cardiovascular disease among AI/AN people and how they can deal with the major risk factors for heart disease:

high blood cholesterol, high blood pressure, overweight and obesity, and physical inactivity. It highlights heart-healthy behaviors to maintain a balance in life and to leave a legacy of health to future generations. In one section, elders from several tribes serve as role models. They describe how they have adopted heart-healthy behaviors and give messages that are simple, heart-felt and powerful. The video is suitable for all tribes and a useful educational tool for clinic waiting rooms, patient groups, community health fairs, and school health classes.

- *Easy to Read Brochures* - In collaboration with Laguna Pueblo in New Mexico, the Ponca Tribe in Oklahoma, and the Bristol Bay Area Corporation in Alaska, the NHLBI created a series of culturally appropriate educational booklets on how to keep a healthy heart. Three sets of booklets were produced, one for each of the tribes listed above. Each set has four brochures in color on practical tips for heart healthy living and contains the following titles: "Your Choice for Change", "Be Heart Healthy! Learn Ways to Lower Your Cholesterol", "Lower Your Blood Pressure! Get Your Blood Pressure Checked Today!", and "Watch Your Weight for a Healthy Heart!"
    - *Honoring the Gift of Heart Health Manual* – the manual provides everything needed to conduct a 10-session educational program on heart health in Native American communities. It is an attractive, easy-to-use, illustrated, leader's guide with skill-building provides AI/ANs the knowledge, skills and motivation to help them take action against heart disease. A CD with visuals in Power Point comes with each manual. Each education session lasts about 2 hours when conducted in the community. The 10 sessions focus on risk factors for CVD and include several sessions that are pertinent to obesity prevention including: Be More Physically Active, Maintain a Healthy Weight, and Make Heart Health Eating a Family Affair. The manual and CD, with separate versions for AIs and ANs are available at: https://www.nhlbi. nih.gov/health-pro/resources/heart/american-indian-health-educator-manual.htm

The second phase of the project has focused on capacity building and community mobilization in tribal communities with intensive education of community and tribal healthcare workers on cardiovascular prevention. In partnership with the IHS Native American Cardiology Program, the

NHLBI, conducted one national workshop and six regional skills-building, train-the-trainer workshops between 2003 and 2006. Over 220 tribal professionals and paraprofessionals have taken part in these workshops, including community health representatives, diabetes educators, health educators, wellness and fitness specialists, and public health nurses. The intent was to have these participants return to their own communities to conduct additional train-the-trainer workshops and to implement Honoring the Gift of Heart Health at the local community level.

The evaluation component of the national and regional train-the- trainer workshops entails assessment of knowledge and awareness of training participants as well as formative and process evaluation measures.

Enthusiasm for this project continues to grow and has stimulated local efforts to promote heart health behavior change in tribal communities. In local tribal communities throughout the U.S., a network of an additional 300 heart health educators have taken part in Honoring the Gift of Heart Health workshops. The IHS Special Diabetes Projects for Indians (SDPI) -CVD Risk Reduction Project Grantees have been using these materials as part of their required intervention activities.

Feedback from tribal communities indicate that the Honoring the Gift of Heart Health is flexible and can be used in a variety of ways; user friendly and easily modifiable; and culturally relevant with regard to food, physical activity and descriptive scenarios related to AI/ANs. Some challenges include: length of each session in a community setting may be too long, making it difficult to recruit and retain community participants; identification of funds to support implementation for train-the-trainer workshops and/or community education sessions; and competing tribal priorities. Some tribal programs have found success with integrating Honoring the Gift of Heart Health into preexisting settings or groups, rather than trying to form new CVD education sessions for community members.

The third phase of the project will focus on clinical and behavioral interventions, by linking community education efforts with the clinical and behavioral outcomes. Partnering with tribes, the IHS and other tribal organizations have been key to the success of Honoring the Gift of Heart Health. Furthermore, the partnership between the NHLBI and IHS demonstrates a successful interagency partnership that can make promising strides towards eliminating health disparities associated with heart disease and stroke.

Healthy Children, Strong Families and Supportive Communities Intervention. The University of Wisconsin-Madison is working in collaboration with the Bad River Tribe, the Lac du Flambeau Tribe, the Menominee Tribe, the Great Lakes Inter-Tribal Council, and the University of New Mexico to conduct a study targeting obesity and CVD prevention. The study is designed to: 1) test the effectiveness of a mentored home-visiting and group support intervention to improve nutrition and physical activity levels in Wisconsin Al preschoolers and their primary caregivers, 2) involve each community in detailed assessments of the macro-level community environmental supports and barriers regarding diet and physical activity, and 3) incorporate participatory research in order to develop culturally acceptable community-based interventions and increase community research capacity. This randomized controlled trial began in FY 2006, and will be implemented over the course of 5 years.

During year 1 of the intervention, targeted home visits will be conducted involving trained Al mentors who will work with 3-5 year old Al children and their primary caregivers to promote skill-based behavior change. During year 2, intervention families will attend monthly group meetings with activities to sustain changes made in Year 1. Control families will receive intervention materials and newsletters only. Seventy-five Al families will comprise each of the two arms of the study. Primary outcomes are decreased child waist circumference and decreased caregiver BMI. Secondary outcomes include: increased fruit/vegetable consumption, decreased TV viewing, increased physical activity, decreased soda/sweetened drink consumption, improved caregiver biochemical indices, and increased caregiver self-efficacy to adopt healthy behaviors. The study utilizes community advisory boards to design and prioritize assessments of food, recreation, economic, legal, and other community systems. These boards will utilize focus groups, surveys, GIS mapping, and direct observation in their evaluations.

Native Healthy Lifestyle: A Return to Balance. The University of Oklahoma Health Science Center working in collaboration with seven tribes in southwest Oklahoma (Apache, Caddo, Comanche, Delaware, Ft. Sill Apache, Kiowa, and Wichita) as well as the Lawton Indian Hospital and the Anadarko Indian Clinic is conducting a randomized controlled trial that will test a holistic behavioral and lifestyle intervention program. This intervention targets 200 AI adults aged 30-59 years who are at high risk of developing CVD and utilizes behavioral modification involving diet and physical activity. The control group will receive conventional cardiovascular health information and advice only. The primary outcome measures will be behavioral modification outcomes, including caloric intake, sodium intake, fruit, and vegetable consumption for diet; and pedometer measurements for physical activity. The secondary outcome measures are CVD risk factors including weight (or BMI), total triglyceride, HDL-cholesterol, LDL- cholesterol, HbA1c, fasting glucose, blood pressure, and urinary albumin/creatinine ratio. This culturally appropriate and community-responsive behavioral intervention program began in FY 2006 and will be implemented over a 5 year period

Healthy Hearts Across Generations. In FY 2006, The University of Washington and the Tulalip Tribes began a 5-year culturally appropriate developmental CVD risk prevention program targeting physical activity levels and food habits among 240 adults who are at high risk for CVD.

The first two phases of the study involve qualitative interviews and a tribal health survey, which will inform the development of the intervention, as well as establish preliminary baseline prevalence rates for self-reported CVD and its correlates. In a 4-month randomized controlled trial, the intervention phase will test an indigenist stress coping model. This model posits that the effect of life stressors (e.g., historical trauma) on health is moderated by cultural factors such as identify attitudes that function as buffers, strengthening emotional health and mitigating the effects of stressors (Walters & Simoni, 2002). Parts of the intervention will include testing NHLBI's *Honoring the Gift of Heart Health* program for AI (described above), talking circles, and individual counseling, all incorporating discussion of historical trauma and interruptions of traditional food supplies. The primary outcome measures are dietary intake and physical activity levels. Secondary outcomes include BMI, fasting glucose, cholesterol, and blood pressure. The study will be conducted over a 5 year period.

Web-based, Patient-centered Approach to CVD Risk-factor Management and Reduction. The Black Hills Center for American Indian Health working in collaboration with the Cheyenne River Sioux Tribe, the University of Washington and the University of Colorado Health Science Center is conducting a randomized controlled trial that will test new home-based, cognitive strategies for CVD prevention among 180 AI adults, 18-69 years of age. The study targets a cohort of AIs, who have been diagnosed with diabetes and hypertension or hypercholesterolemia, but who are free of, but at high risk for CVD and have prescribed physiologic therapies and behavioral instructions that they have been given to manage their CVD risk factors. Goals of this study include improving the adherence of participants by addressing diet, exercise, and smoking and providing them with a culturally-tailored, home health-based chronic disease management program, coupled with the requisite hardware, software, training, and staffing, that will supplement in a paradigm-changing way the route in which they presently receive care. The web-based module will include diabetes training and case management services. Primary outcome measures are glycosylated hemoglobin (HbA1c), blood pressure, and cholesterol. Secondary outcomes include adherence to lifestyle behaviors--diet, smoking, and physical activity. This study began in FY 2006 and will be implemented over a 5 year period,

Key NIH Informants

Karen Donato, NHLIB, Office of the Director, NIH. Van Hubbard, ASPE & NIDDK.

Lisa Gansheroff, NIDDK, Office of the Director, NIH.

Sandy Garfield, NIDDK, Division of Diabetes, Endocrinology & Metabolic Disease, NIH. Phoenix Branch Scientists -- William Knowler MD, Clifton Bogardus, Jonathan Krakoff, Mary Hoskin, Robert Nelson, and Robert Hanson, NIDDK, NIH.

Jared Jobe, NHLIB, Division of Prevention and Population Sciences, NIH. Joan Gallivan, NIDDK, Office of the Director, NIH.

Jane Kelly, Coordinating Center for Health Promotion, CDC. Rachael Tracy, NHLBI, Office of the Director, NIH.

Carla Herman, Professor of Medicine, University of New Mexico.

Centers for Disease Control and Prevention (CDC)

The following CDC activities are described in this section:

- Native Diabetes Wellness Program;
- Eagle Book Series;
- Associate of Science Degree/Diabetes Prevention Specialist Certificate;
- CD Cynergy American Indian/Alaska Native Diabetes Edition;
- Mapping a Shared Vision of Hope;

- Health Promotion and Diabetes Prevention Projects for AI/AN Communities: Adaptations of Practical Community Environmental Indicators;
- Nutrition and Physical Activity Program to Prevent Obesity and Other Chronic Diseases;
- Pediatric Nutrition Surveillance System;
- Pregnancy Nutrition Surveillance System; and
- Well-Integrated Screening and Evaluation for Women Across the Nation (WISEWOMAN) Program

Division of Diabetes Translation (DDT)

Native Diabetes Wellness Program (NDWP). The purpose of the NDWP is to support AI/AN communities in developing effective strategies for care and prevention of diabetes (including obesity prevention) and to develop and sustain alliances with AI/AN and other organizations around this purpose. The NDWP works to reduce the burden of diabetes in the U.S. by combining support for public health-oriented diabetes prevention and control programs (DPCPs) and translating diabetes research findings into widespread clinical and public health practice. In collaboration with IHS, CDC established the National Diabetes Prevention Center (NDPC) located in Gallop New Mexico in 1998. The NDPC supports tribal-specific education systems, diabetes self-management education, and intertribal sharing of diabetes prevention strategies. Key activities of the NDWP are listed below:

- *Diabetes Education in Tribal Schools (DETS) Program.* The lead agency is NIH/NIDDK; collaborating partners and co-funders include CDC and IHS. This project is described in the NIH/NIDDK section of the report.
- *Eagle Book Series.* This book series consists of four diabetes prevention stories for Native American children. These small books are designed for children ages 5-8 and share important messages about diabetes promotion, physical activity, nutrition, and healthy eating. In these stores, a wise eagle assumes the role of tribal elder in the time- honored Native American tradition of using storytelling to pass on tribal culture and to teach the lessons of life. The books will be disseminated to BIA schools as well as schools with 25 percent native enrollment. A teacher's guide and finger puppets that go with three of the books will be included in the packets sent to the schools.

There is no evaluation component; however, a formative evaluation was conducted in the beginning of the project, using focus groups and input from the IHS tribal leaders.

- *Associate of Science (AS) Degree or Diabetes Prevention Specialist Certificate.* This is a new program (in existence for only 6 semesters at the time of this report) that is supported by CDC and the University of New Mexico at Gallup. The purpose of program is to provide academic training in diabetes prevention. CDC has supported a full time coordinator for the program and later a part time coordinator for the program. The Certificate (32 credits) can be obtained by studying part time for a year, while the AS degree (72 credits) involves 2 years of full time study. In May 2006, three students received certificates; one student received an AS. This academic program is the only one of its kind in the U.S., and other schools have expressed an interest in implementing similar programs.

While both native and nonnative students enter these programs, 80% of the students attending the University of New Mexico at Gallup are Native Americans. Most are adult students who are also single parents. If they do not move to Gallup, the students must drive 50 miles each way to and from their reservation to attend class, although classes have also been held on the reservation. Currently thc program has 38 students, and is planning for 20 new students. About half of these students have jobs; for example, in home health care, as school fitness aids or working on diabetes management with elders at senior centers. The remainder of the students have an interest in diabetes; students also take these courses as nursing elective classes.

The curricula includes four basic courses (i.e., Medical Terminology, Basic Anatomy and Physiology, Basic Nutrition, and Health Program Planning), five diabetes courses (i.e., Perspectives in Diabetes, Diabetes Prevention I and II, Diabetes Wellness, and Diabetes Nutrition) and core courses for the AS degree. Native students incorporate their culture into this training by using examples from their own life experiences. Tuition for the Certificate and AS programs is $1472 and $3266 respectively, not including books, travel and miscellaneous expenses.

One faculty member noticed that students were dropping out at the end of the program because of transportation issues. Consequently, she decreased the duration of her courses from 16 to 8 weeks, but increased the amount of time for each session. Student evaluations have indicated that it would be useful to have a specific textbook for the course. Currently, materials are selected from different sources.

As of December 2006, the previous coordinator is supported by CDC through McKing Consulting, Inc. and is working to further the curriculum development by making it amenable to distance learning and community training in addition to classroom participation. Recently the staff of McKing Consulting found that Central Arizona College University has a similar community based program that has been implemented throughout the Southwest, and they are working with that program to integrate the curricula, evaluate progress and outcomes, and determine next steps.

- *CDCynergy American Indian/Alaska Native Diabetes Edition.* This is an interactive training and decision support tool in a CD format that is designed to help conceptualize, plan and develop a health communication program tailored towards diabetes prevention in AI/AN populations. It includes a step-by-step tutorial complete with resources, case studies of health communication methods, a media library, and short discussions by tribal members.
- *Mapping a Shared Vision of Hope.* This public health tool in the form of a CD guides AI/AN communities in developing effective Geographic Information System (GIS) mapping and analysis strategies to display and analyze data for the purpose of developing and evaluating diabetes care and prevention programs in Indian Country. This tool enables the discovery of spatial distributions among health and social variables related to diabetes and other health care issues in AI/AN communities. Custom reports for health disparities, diabetes prevention, and Census data can be created. The CD was developed by the National Indian Council on Aging, Earth Data Analysis Center at the University of New Mexico, and CDC's National Diabetes Prevention Center.
- *Health Promotion and Diabetes Prevention Projects for AI/AN Communities: Adaptations of Practical Community Environmental Indicators (CFDA 93.945).* The purpose of this program supported by the DDT is to strengthen local capacity of AI/AN communities to implement limited, practical community environmental interventions for health promotion and diabetes prevention targeted to a specified population group (e.g., children, young adults, elderly). In September 2005, awards were made to eight tribal communities for simple environmental adaptations; for example, the presence or absence of

low-fat, low-sugar food alternatives in vending machines in public buildings; miles of walking trails per capita; or the proportion of restaurant menu items that follow nutritional guidelines. These awards are in the form of 3 year cooperative agreements -- the first year is a planning grant, and implementation occurs during the second and third years. The grantees are awarded approximately $100,000 per year. Applicants must conduct an evaluation of the community intervention. This is the first time that the DDT has worked directly with tribes; they will offer technical assistance to the grantees.

Division of Nutrition and Physical Activity

Nutrition and Physical Activity Program to Prevent Obesity and Other Chronic Diseases. This is a state-based program whose major goals are balancing caloric intake and expenditure, increasing physical activity, improving nutrition through increased consumption of fruits and vegetables, reducing television time, and increasing breastfeeding. In 2005-2006, 21 states were funded through cooperative agreements at $400,000 - $450,000 for capacity building, and 7 states were funded at $750,000 - $1.3 million for basic implementation, for a total of 28 funded states.

While this program is open to federally recognized tribes, no tribes have applied; thus, all programs serving AI/AN/NAs receive funding through their states. The key informant for this program indicated a need for additional funding specifically for serving tribes and suggested a restricted cooperative agreement for tribes only.

This program uses a social-ecological model and emphasizes a community-based approach. Social marketing techniques are used to assess needs, and community partners determine their own solutions. CDC staff offer training and technical assistance and are involved in site visits. An evaluation component is included; the Research Triangle Institute is the evaluator for all the state programs. Outcomes can involve changes in body mass index (BMI), behavior, policy or the environment.

Although these programs are not specific to tribes, tribal members participate in capacity building and implementation interventions in the following seven states: Montana, New Mexico, New York, North Carolina, Colorado, Massachusetts, and Texas. Interventions vary by state and are described at http://www.cdc.gov/nccdphp/dnpa/obesity/state_ programs/ For example, New Mexico held five regional workshops to identify community needs, gaps and barriers; convened a steering committee to develop the structure of the state plan; held a statewide forum on the state plan; and planned a University of New Mexico Obesity Symposium on Overweight in Children. In addition, an action plan to address nutrition and physical activity in schools (K-12) is being implemented by the New Mexico Action for Healthy Kids Coalition.

The key informant indicated that the trend in these programs is toward *multi-level multi- component interventions* that involve more than one level of the social-ecological model (i.e., societal/media, community, organizational, interpersonal, and individual) as well as more than one key strategy (i.e., physical activity, fruits and vegetables, breastfeeding, portion size, and sweet beverages). For example, in Massachusetts school-based activities involve: 1) integration of nutrition and physical activity into the curriculum of existing core subjects; 2) assessment of nutrition and physical activity policies and systems in schools using CDC's School Health Index; 3) before- and after-school nutrition and physical activity programs; and 4) a campaign in middle schools to promote the 5-2-1 message (i.e., 5 fruits, 2 hours TV/day, and 1 hour active play/day).

Pediatric Nutrition Surveillance System (PedNSS). The Maternal and Child Nutrition Branch of CDC's Division of Nutrition and Physical Activity operate the PedNSS as well as the Pregnancy Nutrition Surveillance System (PNSS) described below. Both systems include AI/ANs among other groups. Both are program-based surveillance systems that monitor the nutritional status of low-income infants, children and women in federally funded maternal and child health programs. CDC contributes funding for the purpose of updating tribal surveillance data systems.

PedNSS data from 2004 represent more than seven million children from birth to age five. A majority of the data are from the Special Supplemental Nutrition Programs for Women, Infants, and Children (WIC) program that serves children up to age 5, although data are also available on children and adolescents up to 20 years of age who receive routine care from public health clinics. Participation by states and tribes is voluntary. The sample includes children in the states submitting data (includes AI/AN children) as well as AI children from the participating tribes.

Available tables show growth indicators (e.g., birth weight, short stature, underweight, overweight, anemia and breastfeeding) for children participating in the WIC program in 2004 by age (0-2 and 2-5 years) and by racial/ethnic group as well as a summary of trends from 1994-2004. Data from the six participating tribes can be compared to state-specific and Nation data. Further detail about PedNSS can be found at: http://www.cdc.gov/pednss/what_is/pednss/

In the 2004 annual PedNSS report, the 6 participating tribes (out of 33 WIC programs) included: InterTribal Council of AZ, Cheyenne River – South Dakota, Chickasaw Nation – Oklahoma, Navajo Nation – Arizona, Rosebud Sioux – South Dakota, and Standing Rock – North Dakota. However, 19 additional tribal WIC programs have WIC information systems that could generate PedNSS data items, and they have expressed an interest in participating in the PedNSS

The key informant indicated that through an interagency agreement with IHS, a new full time Public Health Nutritionist position based in Atlanta will begin in January 2006. This person will assist 19 additional tribes to submit data to the PedNSS and will serve as a focal point for tribal governments participating in the PedNSS and the PNSS by providing technical assistance for collecting, analyzing and interpreting surveillance data; collaborating with the IHS in the development and evaluation of culturally appropriate nutrition and physical activity interventions for the prevention of overweight among AI/AN children; and collaborating with IHS funded epidemiology centers.

The Pregnancy Nutrition Surveillance System (PNSS). In 2004, PNSS data represent approximately 856,123 low income pregnant and postpartum women participating in WIC and the Title V Maternal and Child Health Program. This data includes pre-pregnancy BMI and greater than ideal weight gain during pregnancy in persons from 25 states and the same 6 tribes submitting data to the PedNSS. AI/AN women are included in the state totals, and data pertaining to the six participating tribes is separated out. Available tables show the prevalence of the above health indicators by race/ethnicity in 2004 and also indicate trends by race/ethnicity between 1994-2004. Data from the six tribes can be compared to state and Nation data. Further detail about the PNSS can be found at: http://www.cdc.gov/pednss/what_is/pnss/

Division for Heart Disease and Stroke Prevention

Well-Integrated Screening and Evaluation for Women Across the Nation (WISEWOMAN) Program. In 1993, Congress authorized the Centers for Disease Control and Prevention (CDC) to establish the WISEWOMAN program to extend the services provided within the National Breast and Cervical Cancer Early Detection Program (NBCCEDP) framework. This framework provides the opportunity to target other chronic diseases among women, including heart disease, the leading cause of death among women.

A subset of the women (those who are 40–64 years of age) who participate in NBCCEDP may also participate in WISEWOMAN. The primary purpose of the WISEWOMAN program is to reduce cardiovascular disease and chronic disease risk factors for low-income, uninsured women who may be part of ethnic/minority populations. For additional information, see www.cdc.gov/ wisewoman. Addressing risk factors such as elevated cholesterol, high blood pressure, diabetes, obesity, sedentary lifestyle, atherogenic diet, and smoking can help reduce a woman's risk of cardiovascular disease-related illness and death.

In 1995, CDC launched the first WISEWOMAN demonstration projects in three states: Massachusetts, Arizona, and North Carolina. In 2001, Congress authorized WISEWOMAN to expand to no more than 15 states/tribes. As of 2004, WISEWOMAN reached the cap, with 13 state health departments and 2 tribal organizations receiving funds to provide WISEWOMAN services.

Participants are involved in culturally appropriate lifestyle intervention programs, and they must commit to a certain level of participation and maintenance. The projects use recommendations that support the U.S. Dietary Guidelines and/or the Dietary Approaches to Stop Hypertension (DASH) eating plan. CDC has developed a standard set of minimum data elements that must be collected for all participants at baseline and at the end of one year, and these data are submitted twice annually.

Currently, two of the projects are targeted specifically to Alaska Native women. CDC funds all of the projects at a total of approximately $10 million/year, and funding is available through 2008. Each site uses a different intervention model with a focus on modifying behavioral risk factors. The strengths of the WISEWOMAN program are: 1) targeting of disparate populations and 2) use of the existing NBCCEDP program structure with providers in each state and an intervention that includes collaboration between public health disciplines working in a variety of areas (e.g., diabetes, physical activity, smoking, breast and cervical cancer).

For the purposes of this report, the two projects in Alaska are of special interest. One is implemented by the Southcentral Foundation (SCF), which is included in the Alaska Native Tribal Health Consortium, and the other is carried out by the Southeastern Alaska Regional Health Consortium (SEARHC). Community health workers conduct much of the outreach at both Alaska sites. At both sites, after the screening event (blood, cholesterol, glucose level and other tests), the women are introduced to the core lifestyle intervention curriculum called *Traditions of the Heart*. This curriculum covers nutrition, stress management, exercise, and tobacco use cessation and was adapted from an existing curriculum written at the sixth-grade reading level (University of North Carolina). A lifestyle approach is utilized with the focus on eating healthy foods, engaging in physical activity, making small steps that have an impact, and being a role model for family members.

The SCF effort is research-based, testing the effectiveness of a 12-session group lifestyle intervention using a delayed intervention group that serves as a control group, while the SEARHC program provides 2 intervention sessions with a health educator on an individual basis and evaluates the results of these efforts. In addition, SEARHC women are invited to attend health initiatives and "gatherings." At these gatherings, the women share their stories and help each other maintain their new healthy habits. The SEARHC group tailors its interventions to be culturally relevant to 18 different communities.

Participants in these Alaska programs face challenges including the nature of the weather, residence in small villages, and the cost of healthy food. The SCF found that retention improved if there were fewer sessions held for longer periods. Cultural adaptations include inclusion of culturally appropriate language; use of affordable and available foods commonly eaten in Alaska including traditional food choices; a cookbook with Alaska Native recipes; and exercise lessons adapted to reflect Alaskan activities which are dictated by climate, accessibility, cost and environment.

Two interesting studies pertaining to WISEWOMAN are reported in the literature. One of these-a pilot randomized controlled trial of Alaska Native women at the SCF site (Witmer et al., 2004) is described in the Intervention (Clinical) section of this report.

The other study (Finkelstein et al., 2004) included 5596 WISEWOMAN participants (including 626 ANs from the Alaska programs) and examined racial/ethnic disparities in coronary heart disease risk factors among enrollees. They found that WISEWOMAN participants had a high degree of CVD risk and that there were significant racial/ethnic disparities in risk factors. Among Blacks and Alaska Natives, the average BMI was in the obese range; controlling for individual and community characteristics did not change this result. Additionally, Black participants were at the greatest risk of CVD, while Hispanic and AN participants were healthier in terms of CVD risk than White participants.

In the Finkelstein et al., study, many of the racial/ethnic disparities in CVD risk factors were explained by differences in individual and community characteristics, but other disparities persisted even after controlling for these factors. Some of the community characteristics included in the study were: median earnings of females, racial isolation, proportion of urban population, proportion of female population with high school diploma, income inequality, proportion of families in poverty, number of robbery arrests per 100,000, and population density per square mile. The authors concluded that to be effective, interventions should address community-level factors that may inhibit an individual's ability to undertake specific activities (e.g., crime rates impact opportunity to be physically active) and be tailored to ensure that individuals are able to engage in and benefit from the activities promoted by the intervention.

Key CDC Informants

Dara Murphy, Branch Chief in Division of Diabetes Translation, CDC. Dawn Satterfield, Division of Diabetes Translation, CDC.

Diane Thompson, Nutrition Team Lead in the Maternal Child Nutrition Brach of the Division of Nutrition and Physical Activity, CDC.

Robin Hambre, Team Lead for the Obesity Prevention Programs in the Division of Nutrition and Physical Activity, CDC.

Lemyra Debruyn, Division of Diabetes Translation, CDC.

Susan Anderson, Division of Nutrition and Physical Activity, CDC.

Chris Stockmyer, WISEWOMAN Project Officer, National Center for Chronic Disease

Prevention and Health Promotion, Division of Diabetes Translation, CDC. Rosemary Anslow, Adjunct Professor, University of New Mexico at Gallup

U.S. Department of Agriculture (USDA)

The USDA activities that are described in this section include:

- National Research Initiative: Nutrition and Obesity;
- Seven Generations of Health: A Transgenerational Approach to Human Nutrition and Obesity Intervention in Indian Country;
- Woodlands Wisdom Nutrition Project; and
- Food Distribution Program on Indian Reservations

USDA's National Research Initiative: Human Nutrition and Obesity. Obesity prevention is one of the areas included in this cross-cutting competitive grant program that makes annual awards for research projects and for integrated projects (involving two of three of the following: research, education and extension/outreach objectives). The program is open to a wide variety of organizations – among them the land grant institutions including 33 tribal colleges on the U.S. mainland and 17 such colleges in Alaska and

Hawaii that receive formula funds. Some of the competitive programs are open only to the tribal colleges.

Projects funded by this program are intended to lead to a better understanding of the behavioral and environmental factors that influence obesity and to the development and evaluation of effective interventions to prevent obesity. The 10 year goals for the program include:

- the behavioral and environmental factors that influence obesity will be sufficiently well understood to develop effective obesity prevention strategies;
- valid behavioral and environmental instruments for measuring progress in obesity prevention will be available; and
- effective strategies for preventing overweight and obesity will be available.

One of the priorities for the integrated projects is to target population groups at increased risk for the development of obesity, such as racial and ethnic minorities and those who are economically or educationally disadvantaged. Recently, there have been three AI-related projects involved in this program:

- *Seven Generations of Health: A Transgenerational Approach to Human Nutrition and Obesity Interventions in Indian Country.* This integrated project emphasizes applied or translational research and is described in detail below. At the time of this report, it was the only full competitive grant in this program related to AIs.
- *Woodlands Wisdom Nutrition Project.* Five tribal colleges and the University of Minnesota were involved in creating a 2 year food and nutrition curriculum in which local tribal culture and knowledge interfaces with nutrition science principles. This project is described in more detail below.
- *Turtle Mountain Community College, North Dakota.* USDA is providing bridge funding to this institution to be used for developing a project pertaining to the prevention of type 2 diabetes through physical activity and healthy eating for school-aged children.

Seven Generations of Health: A Transgenerational Approach to Human Nutrition and Obesity Interventions in Indian Country. This project, funded by the Cooperative State Research, Education and Extension Service

(CSREES) at USDA, is a collaborative effort among Native American communities, institutions of higher learning, health agencies, health educators, curriculum specialists and peer educators. Partners include: Southwestern Indian Polytechnic Institute, CDC, IHS, American Indian Research and Education Center at the University of Nevada in Las Vegas, and the Office of Native American Diabetes Program at the University of New Mexico. The project began in August 2004 and is funded for 4 years at $800,000. The project has two primary goals: 1) to develop and disseminate accurate, culturally relevant information about nutrition, exercise and obesity prevention throughout Indian Country and 2) to establish a community-based infrastructure for life-long healthy lifestyles (e.g., *Seven Generations* into the future) in four Native American communities that reflect different populations and generations: Alamo Little Navajo Nation (small isolated reservation near Mexican border), First Nations HealthSource in Albuquerque (urban Indians), Pueblo of Isleta Elderly Center (elderly) and Southwestern Indian Polytechnic Institute (students).

One of the project's primary activities is the evaluation and modification of existing curricula pertaining to nutrition, obesity and diabetes in order to develop a comprehensive curriculum that reflects Native American values and lifestyles. This curriculum will then be used by Native American peer educators in community-based health programs through a Train-the-Trainer approach. These peer educators will also facilitate "Healthy Lifestyle Clubs" (modeled after the old Cooperative Extension clubs) at each of the four sites.

Activities are site-specific, reflecting local needs. A variety of methods are used to deliver health and nutrition content such as: health-related workshops, distance education, activities directed by the peer educators, newsletters, videotapes, a website, and CD-ROMs. For example, at the Southwestern Indian Polytechnic Institute site, a family night was held that offered cooking activities and provided a backpack for children that included the Eagle Book series (described in CDC section of this report). At the Isleta Elderly Center, participants implemented an Intergenerational Traditional Day involving elders and children and other activities for the elderly such as line dancing and gardening. At the Alamo site, breastfeeding education is a focus as well as team participation in a "Walk Across New Mexico" activity.

An outside evaluator will evaluate this project utilizing both qualitative and quantitative methods. Rather than weight loss, the outcomes of interest are: participation in the site activities, culturally relevant curricula and activities, and creation of a durable infrastructure in the sites that will sustain these activities. The final report will include a replicable model for the Healthy Lifestyle Clubs.

Woodlands Wisdom Nutrition Project. The concept for this project originated because of the dilemma that although AI communities suffer disproportionately from several diet-related chronic diseases, they remain underrepresented within the nutrition and dietetics professions. Representatives from tribal colleges across the upper Midwest worked together and invited the University of Minnesota to become an equal partner. The project involved the creation of a cross-cultural food and nutrition curriculum where local tribal culture and knowledge interfaces with nutrition science principles. The four key objectives of the project were: 1) to increase the number of Native American practitioners in nutrition and food science; 2) to identify and research the relationship of diet to health; 3) to increase community engagement with issues of food and health; and 4) to create a mechanism to network throughout the region.

The project resulted in the Woodlands Wisdom Food and Nutrition Associate of Science Degree Program (includes 55 credit hours of required courses) that was approved by each of the participating tribal colleges. The curriculum is fully described in Hassel's (2006) article. Students graduating from this program may proceed to work toward becoming registered dieticians. The project seeks to shift attention from the visible and tangible levels of artifacts and objects (foods) to the underlying worldviews and knowledge systems that are less visible, but more powerful in terms of guiding AI cultural practices. Evaluation data pertaining to student outcomes were not yet available. However, studies from Canada indicate that indigenous students can experience greater success in the sciences when courses are grounded within an appropriate cultural worldview orientation.

Food Distribution Program on Indian Reservations (FDPIR). FDPIR provides commodity foods (examples provided below) to low income households living on Indian reservations and to AI households residing in approved areas near reservations or in Oklahoma. Many households participate in the FDPIR as an alternative to the Food Stamp Program (FSP) because they do not have easy access to FSP offices or authorized food stores. Households are prohibited from participating in FDPIR and the FSP at the same time.

FDPIR is administered at the federal level by USDA's Food and Nutrition Service (FNS) and at the local level by either Indian Tribal Organizations (ITOs) or an agency of a state government. Currently, 257 tribes in 22 states are utilizing this program. In FY 2006, $82.5 million was appropriated for FDPIR. This includes the federal share of local administrative costs and 100 percent of the food purchases. FDPIR is implemented at the request of the tribes; some tribes choose not to take part in this program. Reasons for this may include low numbers of potentially eligible households due to tribal per capita payments and lack of resources or infrastructure to support the program.

FDPIR offers only products that are grown and processed in the U.S. or its territories. The list of available foods does not include highly perishable items such as fresh fluid milk or fresh eggs. Participants may select from over 90 products each month, including frozen ground beef; frozen cut-up chicken; canned meats, poultry, and fish; flour; cornmeal; bakery mix; reduced sodium crackers; macaroni and cheese; pastas; cereals; rice; juices; fresh and caned fruits and vegetables; canned and dry beans; canned soups; spaghetti sauce; egg mix; vegetable oil, butter; cheese; milk products; and peanuts and peanut butter.

A review workgroup, consisting of representatives from the ITOs, state agencies, FNS Regional Offices, tribal health systems, CDC, and IHS, meets periodically to review the foods that are offered under FDPIR. In each review cycle, the workgroup develops its own goals and makes recommendations to FNS. The members of the workgroup may change each review cycle to reflect different regional perspectives.

Discussions with key FDPIR staff provided basic information on program oversight, program strengths and challenges, best practices, and directions for future research. With regard to FDPIR's strengths, FNS continues to work to improve program access and customer service to participants. Some of the improvements are listed below:

- Through the years, FNS and its tribal partners have worked to improve the food package by reducing sodium, fat and sugar in the commodities, providing frozen meats as an alternative to canned meats, and introducing foods that appeal to participants. The food package review work group is helping to continue these improvements to the food package.
- Under a contract with the Department of Defense (DoD), ITOs and State agencies may opt to offer fresh produce to participants. DoD purchases and delivers the fresh produce to the programs, allowing households to select from a variety of fresh fruits and vegetables in lieu of canned products. The Fresh Produce initiative began in 1996 and is continuing to expand to more programs. In FY 2006, 90 percent

of the ITOs and State agencies were enrolled in this program. FNS continues to work with those remaining programs to bring them on board. For example, the Navajo Nation is in the process of installing coolers in all of its warehouses and is expected to soon be able to offer fresh produce to its participants.

- Another improvement to the program involves FNS' efforts to expand the number of products with commercial labels. Previously, FNS required generic USDA labels on all products in an effort to control theft and misuse of USDA donated commodities. However, some participants incorrectly perceived products with generic labels as being of lesser quality. FNS is working with the vendors to ensure that more products with commercial labels are offered under FDPIR.
- An Automated Inventory System (AIS), developed by FNS for use in FDPIR, tracks inventory from receipt in the local warehouse to household issuance. AIS also houses certification data, thus allowing the ITOs and State agencies to easily generate all program reports.
- Nutrition education materials are available on the USDA/FNS website. USDA also has an extensive Food and Nutrition Information Center that includes nutrition resource materials that are available to ITOs, State agencies, and the general public.

Below are some examples of FDPIR best practices at the local level:

- Some ITOs have adopted an innovative issuance system whereby participants can select commodities from shelves in a grocery store setting. The selections are validated at a checkout counter to ensure that a household does not exceed its allowable level of commodities. This store concept is very popular among some participants.
- ITOs and State agencies within regions have collaborated and pooled their allocations of FDPIR nutrition education funding to produce region-wide nutrition education materials, including videos on food safety and food handling, recipe books, and calendars highlighting nutrition education.

FDPIR is faced with some key challenges, some of which are also referred to in the Feingold et al. (2005) study discussed in the Nutrition and Diet section of this report.

- Monthly participation has declined over the past several years. Despite recent improvements, average monthly participation in FY 2006 dropped to 89,867, a 36 percent decline from the FY 1987 peak of 140,231, and 30 percent below the more recent average monthly participation peak of 129,466 in FY 1999. Because, this issue has not been carefully studied, the factors contributing to the decline are not clear (USDA, National Data Bank).
- Vendors must undergo a certification process to be able to sell commodities to USDA. For this and other reasons, some vendors choose to not do business with the federal government. This has created a challenge for USDA in buying specific products that are available in the commercial market when the vendor does not participate in the USDA commodity purchase program.

  Additionally, some minority and small business vendors that are awarded a contract for the purchase of commodities do not process products under their own commercial label. Consequently, these vendors must use the USDA generic label. This has created a challenge for USDA in its efforts to expand the number of products with commercial labels.
- There are logistical issues involved in purchasing commodities from the vendors and ensuring that those commodities are delivered to remote tribal locations in a timely manner. USDA purchases products in full truck loads. However, many of the local programs need the products in quantities too small to allow direct shipments (i.e., full truck loads) from the vendor. This means that products must be delivered by the vendor to a central warehouse where orders from the local programs are filled and packed onto a delivery truck (i.e., multi-food shipments). FNS is implementing a new simplified system for the ordering and delivery of multi-food shipments that will reduce the time between placing an order and delivery and improve customer service in terms of guaranteed delivery time frames and ease of ordering.
- Local programs are required to provide nutrition education to program participants. FDPIR appropriations do not earmark funds for nutrition education activities; however, FNS sets aside a portion of each year's appropriation for this purpose. FNS recognizes the need for more directed and collaborative nutrition education efforts at the local level.

While nutritious products are available (e.g., whole wheat flour and low-fat cheese), participants may not know the best ways to incorporate these products into their diets.

The President's FY 2007 budget would provide $1 million dollars for nutrition education in FDPIR. FNS hopes to use these funds to initiate sustainable collaborative FDPIR Nutrition Education Programs similar in concept to the Food Stamp Nutrition Education grant program. ITOs and state agencies would be requested to develop plans for behaviorally-focused interventions that follow the Food Stamp Nutrition Education Guiding Principles. They would be encouraged to create partnerships or collaborations with USDA's Cooperative State Research, Education and Extension Service; State Departments of Health or Education; state-level nutrition networks; the IHS Division of Diabetes Prevention and Control; or others for FDPIR nutrition education services.

- Although FNS has received requests for more traditional foods in the FDPIR food package, some of these foods are costly and do not offer improved nutritional value compared to similar products currently offered under the program. For example, blue corn meal does not offer a significant increase in nutritional value in comparison to the yellow corn meal that is currently provided under FDPIR. However, its cost is quite high compared to the yellow corn meal. Another concern with some traditional foods is the availability of the product in sufficient quantities to serve the entire program. Bison meat, which USDA purchased for FDPIR under special appropriations from FY 2001 to FY 2006, has proven to be difficult to purchase in sufficient quantities.

Key USDA Informants

Dr. Joan Goodman, Southwestern Indian Polytechnic Institute

Etta Saltos, National Program Leader, Competitive Programs, Cooperative State Research, Education and Extension Service, USDA.

Nancy Theodore, Food and Nutrition Service, Food Distribution Program on Indian Reservations, USDA.

Dawn Aldridge, Food Assistance Programs, USDA.

III. SITE VISIT TO GILA RIVER INDIAN COMMUNITY

The purpose of the visit to the Gila River Indian Community on January 26, 2006 was to talk to staff familiar with the various types of obesity treatment and prevention activities that are ongoing for children and/or adults and to observe any of these activities. Information to be gathered included: (1) the nature of the activities, (2) the effectiveness of the activities, and (3) general perceptions about factors involved in the obesity issue. The information gleaned from this site visit is illustrative only of the Gila River Indian Community and cannot be generalized to apply to any other tribes.

Interviewees

Three separate sessions were held. The first of these was conducted with nine staff from the tribal Health Corporation. The second session was held with a representative from the tribe's Department of Human Resources. The final session was held with six researchers from NIH's National Institute of Diabetes and Digestive and Kidney Diseases (NIDDK) based in Phoenix who traveled to Gila River for the meeting. The site visitor was also taken on a tour of the hospital and during this time brief interviews were held with a physical therapist and exercise physiologist.

Background Information

The Gila River Indian Community is located 40 miles south of Phoenix, Arizona and its reservation covers a land area of 581.1 square miles. Its population (2000 Census) is 11,257 and the tribe has 19,266 enrolled tribal members. The Community is composed of the Pima and Mariciopa Tribes and is divided into seven districts that are located in peripheral areas of the Phoenix metropolitan area. The visit took place in District #3, also called Sacaton.

The Community has a diverse economic base that includes Gila River farms, sand and gravel operations, three industrial parks, and three casino/resorts. However, even with these enterprises, poverty and unemployment rates are high. Gaming proceeds go directly to the tribe for the development of their infrastructure rather than to individual tribal members.

Housing is available if income criteria are met. There is a high truancy rate among the youth.

Most tribes have a Health Department as part of their tribal government; however, the Gila River Indian Community formed a 501c(3) tribal Health Corporation.. This quasi-private sector model allows a more autonomous and independent relationship with the tribe, as the Corporation is not dependent on tribal procurement and personnel practices. The Health Corporation employs 700 persons and includes a hospital that has an in-patient unit. The Gila River Indian Community also has other corporations both nonprofit and for profit (e.g., sand and gravel endeavor and casinos). The Health Corporation's budget is supported by: IHS -- 38%, grants 5-6%, and third party revenues (e.g., Medicare, private pay/Blue Cross, Medicaid).

The Gila River Indian Community has taken over operation of a number of IHS programs under self-governance compacts. Tribal services are organized in the following manner: 1) Alcohol and Drug Services, 2) Tribal Department of Public Health, 3) Health Corporation, and 4) Environmental Health Funds. The tribe has its own renal dialysis center, behavioral mental health facility, and is building government and long term care centers. The tribe and the Corporation meet to address issues related to service duplication and sharing of resources.

The Gila River Indian Community has a very high rate of diabetes. Furthermore, at Gila River, over the past 10 years, there has been an increase in cancer rates -- kidney and colon cancer for males and ovarian cancer for women. We know that obesity increases the risk of mortality for adults of all races from colon cancer in men (NRCCDH, 1989). At the Health Corporation, there is a campaign to increase employee leadership through mentorship programs involving the following components of the organization: Information Technology, Managed Care, Business, and Clinical Facilities.

Food Availability

There is only one food market on the reservation, and some food is available at gas station/convenience shops. Tribal members must travel 15-20 miles to reach a grocery store other than the food market referred to above, and this involves transportation costs. It is easier to go to the street vendors who sell unhealthy food such as fry bread. There are no fast food restaurants on the reservation, but they located are nearby. Some tribal members have no refrigerators, electricity or running water.

The Federal Distribution Program on Indian Reservations (FDPIR) has been available on the reservation for 30 years. Fresh produce is available through this program as well as from the tribe's seasonal grapefruit and citrus crops. Respondents mentioned Food Stamps, WIC, and food banks as additional sources of food supplies. Sugared sodas have been removed from vending machines in the Health Corporation. No information was provided about vending machines in the schools.

Recreational Facilities

In Sacaton, the main town on the reservation, there is a hospital-based wellness center (discussed below) and a community wellness center. Tribal members (self or referred) can attend the community wellness center where monthly walks and community programs are held. Programs held at this center have had higher participation than those at the hospital. Respondents indicated that tribal members trust the person leading these activities. Sacaton also has a community gym that has exercise equipment and intramural sports activities for young persons; the extent of their participation was not reported.

The tribe built a community recreation center in District #6 that serves a population of about 4,000 and is located in the west end of the community, 40 miles from Sacaton. This center has an Olympic size swimming pool, but the pool is not being utilized because only one person passed the Red Cross certification necessary to be a lifeguard, and lifeguards are needed to operate this pool.

Attitudes about Obesity

Some respondents indicated that overweight is accepted among community members. Someone who is skinny is perceived as not doing well. If someone is thin, others will say, "You need to fatten up" or ask them "Are you OK?" Other respondents indicated that the culture prizes largeness. Being big is a part of one's identity and is equated with any of the following: being healthy, a good farmer, a sign of wealth, or sexual attractiveness. Respondents did not currently know of any tribal members with eating disorders such as anorexia.

Psychosocial Issues

Respondents identified psychosocial issues as primary barriers to participation in obesity programs; for example, deaths of community members; unresolved grief; poverty; abuse including sexual abuse and domestic violence; substance abuse including alcoholism and a high rate of crystal methamphetamine use; intergenerational conflicts arising from grandparents raising grandchildren; and Sacaton's location between two metro areas and along the Mexican border.

Resource and Other Barriers

Many people have no cars. There are long distances between the various sections of the reservation e.g., 35 miles. The tribe has four vans, but there are a large number of people who need transportation, and thus van service is not always available for self-referrals -- those who might want to go to the community wellness center who are not elderly or on Medicaid.

Childcare resources are also lacking. The tribe has only one childcare center. It is leased to a private company, but it is full and reserved for low income families.

Confidentiality issues were also raised as a barrier to receiving services. Because tribal members are concerned that everyone else will know about their problems or see them in the therapy waiting room, therapy groups are not popular, however, educational groups have greater participation.

Intervention Programs

SuPuKum Ke Wellness Program -- Hospital-Based Wellness Center. This program began in 1999 as a hospital-based Physical Therapy Department. IHS Special Diabetes grant money was used for equipment and staffing. The Wellness Center opened in April of 2001. The target population includes persons who are at risk of diabetes in addition to those at higher medical risk (due to other conditions) who may find it unsafe to use local community-based exercise programs. Persons who do not meet these criteria are encouraged to use the Community Wellness Centers in District 3 or 6.

The Physical Therapy Department has three physical therapists, and the hospital-based Wellness Center has one exercise physiologist, two peer fitness workers, one supervisor, and one van driver. Van service to all seven districts is provided several times per week. Most of the participants in the Wellness Center are previous physical therapy clients. Intake assessments are not done because most of the information needed is included in the medical referral. Although many of the client's problems are obesity-related, center staff does not a focus on weight loss.

Data that was provided for 2001- July 2004 indicated that Wellness Center usage has increased every year since 2001. As of 2004, 45 individuals had been *active* for at least 18 months. The average HbA1c [a lab test that shows the average amount of sugar (also called glucose) in a person's blood over the last 3 months indicating if blood sugar level is normal or too high] at baseline was 8.2%, and the average HbA1c after 18 months was 6.6%. (a HBA1c < 7.0% is associated with the lowest risk of diabetic complications). Most clients are able to reduce their HBA1c by 1% or more after being physically active for 6 months. Clients overwhelmingly reported improvements in their quality of life, and most clients are able to reduce their risk of diabetic complications after being physically active for 6 months.

At the Wellness Center, there are approximately 1400 total wellness visits per month, and community-based exercise classes average 130 visits per month. However, many participants drop out of the Wellness Center. One reason for the dropouts cited by staff is a tendency among participants to deny or ignore health problems.

Thoak Thag Ke Life Center **–** This Center includes two programs – Diabetes Education and the Diabetes Prevention Project. Both programs employ a behavioral health intervention model.

Diabetes Education Program – This program has been ongoing since 2004 and serves those diagnosed with diabetes. The program includes the following components: Diabetes Education, Case Management, Psychology, Physical Activities, and Transportation. In addition to staff working in these components, there is an exercise specialist and clinical abstractor. There are about 2,000 enrollees; 80% are overweight (have a BMI>85%), and 62% are obese. It is not clear how many of those diagnosed with diabetes on the reservation are enrolled or actively involved.

The program offers sessions of various lengths: 1 session , 4 sessions over 4 weeks, and 16 sessions over 16 weeks. Two curricula were mentioned: American Diabetes Association curriculum and the Lifestyle Balance curriculum (used in the Diabetes Prevention Program discussed in the

Intervention section of this report) that includes healthy eating components and physical activity for weight loss as well as one-on-one visits. Diabetes visits are tracked through IHS clinic and hospital data.

Staff described their approach as focusing on health improvement versus weight loss and on small life style changes that people will need to employ for the rest of their lives versus "dieting." Although participants are willing to exercise, they may believe that they can eat what they want after physical activity. Thus, staff try to reinforce the idea that diet and exercise go together. Some staff said that it may not be safe to walk around the reservation, so staff advise: "Walk with a partner."

With regard to weight loss, staff talk about emotional eating. Tribal members give excuses saying that healthy foods involve greater cost or watching one's weight means having to cook meals separately from the family meal. When tribal members experience life issues that interfere with weight loss, staff acknowledged that these issues may interfere with intervention efforts. There have been a few successful cases. Support by case manager and health provider is needed. Mindset and readiness are key factors, but program retention is a problem. Hospital staff indicated their interest in motivational interviewing, and they have invited a nationally recognized expert in this area to come to the reservation to speak.

Diabetes Prevention Program (DPP). This competitive grant is a 5-year demonstration of NIDDK's Diabetes Prevention Program (DPP) designed to translate the results of the DPP research into practice (DPP discussed in Intervention section of this report). At the time of the site visit, the program was in its second year; the first year was a planning grant. The target population is non-diabetic Gila River Indian Community residents at least 18 years of age who have impaired glucose tolerance (IGT) or pre-diabetes. Staff were beginning to do screening and recruiting at district community service meetings, clinical settings, and community activities as well as through the use of advertisements, mailings, and referrals.

The DPP goal for each individual is to lose 7 percent of their weight and to engage in physical activity at least 150 minutes/week. The intervention involves a series of 16 weekly group sessions (within 6 months of joining), one weekly group meeting, and individualized support through case manager intervention. Participants must be willing to stay in the program for 3 years. The DPP is based at Hu Hu Kam Memorial Hospital, but sessions will be conducted at many district service centers. Home visits will be made and transportation can be provided. The program goal is to have 48 adults/year complete the intervention, but in order to meet this goal they must recruit more than this number.

Community-Based Intervention Approaches. In September 2005, the tribe's Human Resources Department began to formulate a new public health approach. Rather than diabetes or obesity (terms implying a medical problem), the focus will be on taking small steps toward physical fitness for health and well being, decreasing risk factors, and "movement" for the sake of sociability. The issue is how to get tribal members to participate, and this involves marketing. There are plans to move the wellness centers located in each of the seven districts closer to the community stations in all seven districts i.e., "stationing resources for access." The tribal key informant believed that if they could get those with diabetes to go for a nightly walk, this would produce better results than anything else. Health Corporation staff also indicated that they would like to see the whole community become actively involved in exercising through a "community campaign." The following two community-based programs were described:

Genesis. This program for parents of children 0-5 years of age has been operational for 5-6 years. The birth rate is 311 per year at the Gila River Indian Community. The emphasis of this program is on overweight infants (e.g., 9 pounds or more at birth) as well as breastfeeding, parental role in diet, skill building, meal preparation, and education about risk factors. The goal is for children to be breastfed for 6 months. The program is based on NIH research findings and started as a result of a DHHS/IHS grant.

Staff indicated that every pregnant woman should be visited by a lactation specialist during her pregnancy; however, it was not clear how many of these mothers are actually visited. The staff includes one nutritionist and four diabetes prevention specialists who are tribal members. Intervention takes place in the home. Each lactation specialist has a caseload of 86, and the follow-up period is 5 years. The weight and height ratios of the children are tracked and grouped into three categories: those at risk, those over 92% of ideal weight, and those underweight. The key informant did not have data on whether breastfeeding rates have increased as a result of the program.

Health Educators. A health prevention program that involves the general population began in May 2005. The staff includes a director, two degreed tribal health educators, and four tribal lay people. These staff will take information on prevention (e.g., obesity and diabetes) into tribal members' homes while using terminology that tribal members can understand. For example, diabetes would be described as, "spilling of sugar" or "urine gets to be sweet." The health educators are focusing on understanding how the tribal members learn and remember; for example, materials that utilize the five senses may facilitate learning for those in this community. The health educators are also studying advertising approaches.

Challenges include: 1) accepted etiquette among tribal members is that people do not enter other people's homes – this is perceived as aggressive; 2) obesity is an accepted lifestyle; 3) understanding the factors that motivate tribal members to remain overweight; and 4) the stigma involved in help-seeking in the tribal community.

School Based Programs -- The schools located on the reservation are measuring BMI and doing glucose testing on a regular basis. Information obtained during the site visit indicated that in order to increase the emphasis on physical education, the tribe has placed full time physical education teachers in four schools for several years.

Ideas for Future Research Provided by Corporation Staff

Health Corporation staff suggested the following areas for future research: 1) prevention of obesity in children; 2) behavior and lifestyle changes; 3) changes in the mentality of the tribe as well as in each person (i.e., emphasing physical activity and utilization of programs); 4) the use of bariatric intervention and its effectiveness for Native Americans; 5) the feasibility of offering obesity programs when overweight is accepted; 6) the issue of a lack of safe areas for walking.

NIDDK Research Presentations

Researchers from NIH's NIDDK Branch located in Phoenix traveled to Gila River to present the following research studies involving Gila River tribal members:

Gila River Indian Community Longitudinal Health Study 1965-: Since 1965, a longitudinal study pertaining to diabetes and its complications has been conducted in a geographically- defined part of the Gila River Indian Community. Approximately every 2 years, each resident of the study area who is at least 5 years old is invited for a biennial health examination. Time trends of median BMI for men and women indicated that for men of most age groups, median BMI has increased over the three time periods: 1965-68, 1983-86, and 2001-2004, and, for women the findings were similar. Furthermore, the incidence of diabetes in adult Pima Indians (who are part of the Gila River Indian Community) increases as BMI increases. Recent analyses suggest that despite the rising BMI over time, the actual incidence of type 2 diabetes in the Gila River Indian Community has remained stable over the last 30 years (Knowler et al., 1990; Kriska et al., 2003).

Diabetes Prevention Project (DPP): Gila River tribal members participated in this multicenter randomized clinical trial (1996-2001) with long term follow-up. The results of this study are fully described in the Intervention section of this report. In all ethnic groups, lifestyle intervention and treatment with metformin both reduced the incidence of diabetes in persons at high risk, and the lifestyle intervention was more effective than metformin (DPP Research Group, 12/2002 and 2/2002).

Look AHEAD (Action for Health in Diabetes)**:** This is a multicenter randomized clinical trial taking place from 2001-2012 in the U.S., and it includes the Gila River Indian Community. The primary objective is to assess the long term effects (up to 11.5 years) of an intensive weight loss program targeted for 4 years to overweight and obese individuals who have type 2 diabetes, are 45-74 years of age, and have a body mass index >25kg/m2. Participants will be randomized into two groups – one will receive intensive lifestyle intervention and one will receive diabetes support and education. The hypothesis is that weight loss can prevent or delay the cardiovascular complications of type 2 diabetes. Federal sponsors include NIDDK, NHLBI, National Institute of Nursing Research (NINR), CDC and others (The Look Ahead Research Group, 2004).

Why some people are obese? The researcher presenting on this topic said that the environment explains differences in weight between populations with similar genetic backgrounds who are living in different environments (e.g., Pima tribes in U.S. are heavier than those Pimas in Mexico), while genetics can help explain differences in weight within populations living in a similar environment (e.g., Pima Indians living in the Southwest U.S.). He indicated that a variety of studies conducted on non-Indians involving twins reared apart, siblings, and adopted twins have found a genetic factor in obesity. The results of his research indicate that two-thirds of the determinants of body weight in Pima Indians (living in the Gila River Indian Community) are due to genetic factors identified as genetic causes for inactivity and genetic causes for hyperphagia. However, to date, some research has not found genetic causes for physical inactivity. He also stated that people have difficulty believing that genetic factors are primary in obesity. In summary, from his perspective, some of the Pima Indians (but not all) have a genetic predisposition to obesity, and this predisposition may interact with environmental factors.

He found that heritability estimates of overweight in the Gila River Indian Community population are high for BMI and percent body fat. He has studied the metabolic rate in Gila River residents, but found this not to be a significant factor in obesity; however, this finding has not been reproduced in other populations. He is now trying to identify susceptibility genes for obesity and type 2 diabetes. He indicated that a genetic MC4R protein structure contributing to obesity has been found, but this occurs only in 5% of the very obese.

Obesity Presentation. Obesity is determined by energy balance: including energy-in (food intake) versus energy-out (metabolism, activity, and waste). On the energy-in side, there is a hormone called ghrelin that rises before meals and causes a desire to eat. In Pimas who gained weight, researchers have found higher levels of ghrelin. On the energy-out side, researchers are studying waste (e.g., nutrient absorption) to see if obese individuals absorb more food than lean individuals, and whether bacteria in the intestine are responsible for these differences. This study is just beginning and to date, there are no findings to report.

The researcher indicated that in most weight loss programs, there are varying levels of success, even in the DPP. Previous studies suggest that how an individual's energy expenditure (metabolism) responds to overfeeding and fasting, may predict how much weight they gain. Based on this response (or phenotype), an NIDDK Obesity Phenotype Intervention Study is currently under consideration. This study will focus on the determinants of success in weight loss programs by characterizing each individual according to how their energy expenditure responds to a short period of overfeeding and underfeeding. Other possible predictors of weight loss will also be measured in this study. This study will enroll approximately 150 individuals, and at least half of the volunteers may be Native American. There will be no control group. All participants will receive a dietary intervention which will be a 25 percent reduction in calories based on what they need to maintain their current weight. Some of the individuals will be asked to remain as inpatients at a clinical research unit for up to 12 weeks for carefully monitored diet plans, while the rest will be followed as outpatients. Prior to the intervention, all participants will spend 2-3 weeks in the hospital for an energy-in evaluation (food intake and hormones), an energy-out evaluation and a psychological evaluation.

The goal of this study is to find predictors of who will be more successful at losing weight and keeping it off. There will be long-term follow-up of at least 4 years after the acute intervention phase and longer if possible. The study will also be able to test how people respond to certain diets or medications. This study is planned to begin in fall 2007, but this depends upon approval processes and protocol development. Although participants will be compensated, involving persons who will follow through with this program will be challenging.

General Discussion with NIDDK Staff

The following issues were brought up in a general discussion with the NIDDK researchers after the presentations discussed above:

- Cultural issues with tribes may involve snakes, heat, taboos against walking, and parents' perceptions of whether their children are overweight.
- Urban Indians may be more familiar with weight loss interventions than tribal members living on the reservations.
- It was noted that there is much more interest among the tribal community in losing weight now versus 30 years ago. Charelton Wilson did a phone survey about weight among urban AIs and found that a high percentage had attempted to lose weight.
- Current studies focus on short-term results versus long-term maintenance of weight loss. This is an area that needs further research.
- In order to look at prevention of obesity, one would have to study a nonobese population over time to see if weight gain could be prevented.
- There are no major differences in the average American diet and the Gila River Indian Community diet as estimated from food purchase data (Knowler et al., 1990). However, there may be cost differences. One survey found that people who perceived their diet was Indian versus Anglo were healthier regardless of what their diet actually was.

Key Informants at Gila River Indian Community

Carol Schurz
Lisa Hussey
Della Acunia-Sockyma
Loren Ellery
Shawn Johnson
Susanne Girard
Monica Martinez
Cheryl Morning
Alphonso Bitsuie
Helen Connor
Evelyn Bird
Henry Walden
Lisa Hussey
Steve Schoffstall

Key Informants from NIDDK in Phoenix

William Knowler
Clifton Bogardus
Jonathan Krakoff
Mary Hoskin
Robert Nelson
Robert Hanson

IV. Directions for Future Research

Research pertaining to obesity and AI/ANs is limited; thus, additional studies are needed in almost every area impacting this topic. The following are the research gaps or unanswered questions that have become apparent as a result of this literature review and discussions with key informants.

Prevalence

- *Longitudinal Studies.* Existing studies indicate that overweight and obesity are significantly higher for AI/AN preschool children, school-aged children and adults compared to U.S. all race national averages.

However, many of these studies are cross- sectional. Longitudinal studies especially of preschool and school-aged children are needed to determine growth patterns over time so that critical intervention points can be identified.

- *Regional Differences.* Existing studies have shown that there are regional differences in the prevalence of obesity for AI/AN children and adults, but the question remains as to what factors contribute to these differences.
- *Urban Indians.* Although, approximately two-thirds of AIs live in urban areas, there is a paucity of research pertaining to the prevalence of obesity in this population.
- *Surveillance Systems.* Improved surveillance systems need to be established in order to monitor growth in AI/AN children, to document the age-specific prevalence rates for overweight and obesity, and to track progress in decreasing obesity at the population level. This data needs to be reported and shared with tribal communities and tribal health departments.

Nutrition and Diet

- *Urban Indians.* Because existing studies focus on reservation-based samples, there is little research on the adequacy of nutrition and diet among urban Indians, and how this compares with those living on or near reservations.
- *Nutrition education.* While nutritious products are available to the tribes through the Food Distribution Program on Indian Reservations (FDPIR), without nutrition education, tribal members may not know the best ways to utilize these or other products. How can the FDPIR most effectively deliver nutrition education to tribes? Could increased coordination between USDA food assistance programs and TANF, IHS and economic development programs of the Bureau of Indian Affairs improve participation, access, availability, and effectiveness of nutrition education?
- *Professional Nutrition Services.* It is estimated that the current number of registered dieticians who work for the Indian Health Service or tribal or urban Indian health programs can currently provide nutrition services to only approximately 15 percent of the

AI/AN population or about 207,000 individuals (IHS, 2001). How can this gap best be filled?

- *Food Stamps (FS) and FDPIR Programs.* Among AI/ANs, who are the consumers of the Food Stamp and FDPIR programs? What are their demographics? Why has the participation rate in FDPIR decreased over recent years? What are the criteria for participants selecting FSP vs. FDPIR, and what are the dynamics of people cycling between the two programs? (Currently, USDA's Economic Research Service is supporting a study that is comparing the FDPIR and the FSP with regard to eligibility, participation, administration and outcomes on health and nutrition).
- *Nutrition and Physical Activity Patterns.* One suggestion by a key informant who contributed to this report was to conduct a pilot study that would survey children and parents involved in IHS' Special Diabetes Program for Indians (SDPI) regarding diet and physical activity behaviors at home and at school. SDPI staff might be involved in administering such a survey, and findings could be used to design effective educational intervention strategies for parents and children.
- *Food Insecurity.* What is the relationship between food insecurity and obesity in AI/AN communities?
- *Lifestyle Changes.* A study could explore the continuum regarding traditional and non- traditional lifestyles for AI/AN individuals/ families. For example, when people become more urban, employed and sedentary (e.g., Alaska Natives who move from a small village to a larger village to a regional hub), what happens to their gathering and use of subsistence foods and their ability to be physically active?
- *Traditional Foods.* The cost of traditional foods for the FDPIR is often prohibitive due to low demand. How can tribes increase the demand for and use of traditional foods to make them more affordable?
- *Food Sharing.* Food is an important part of Native American culture, and the giving of food is important. How does the utilization of food assistance programs interact with tribal norms, such as the sharing of food?
- *Breastfeeding.* What are breastfeeding rates among AI/ANs compared to other groups, and how can these rates be increased?
- *Food Contamination in Traditional Foods.* How do communities/regions (e.g., Alaska Natives) feel about bioloading

contaminants in food, eating contaminated foods, and working in industries that package these foods for others (e.g., mercury in fish)?

Psychosocial Factors

- *Stress.* We know that there are many psychosocial stressors that AI/AN community members experience. What are the cultural buffers (e.g., identity attitudes, enculturation, traditional health practices) that may moderate the vulnerability of AI/ANs in regard to stress (Walters & Simoni, 2002)? What is the relationship between stressors and obesity? How does historical trauma interact with more proximal stressors to exacerbate their effects?
- *Mental Illness.* What is the relationship in AI/AN adults and children between mental illness and/or depression and obesity?
- *Psychological Factors.* What are key psychological factors impacting obesity in AI/ANs; for example, the development of self-esteem, self-efficacy, and resiliency?
- *Environmental Factors.* What are the key environmental factors that influence obesity among AI/ANs including socioeconomic factors and policies (i.e., laws, regulations, informal rules, and practices adopted to guide individual and collective behavior; tribal government acts; and local ordinances)?
- *Perception/Attitudes about Obesity.* A common belief is that American Indian people view overweight/obesity as culturally acceptable or inevitable and therefore are not motivated by health education efforts that focus on preventing or reducing obesity. How true is this belief today among AI/A children and adults in various tribes?

Genetics

- *Interaction of Genetics and Environment.* Continued research is needed to examine genetic factors in AI/ANs, particularly the interaction between genetic and environmental factors.

Intervention Research

Theory and Research Design

- *Improved Theories.* Additional theories on how behavioral and environmental factors influence AI/AN obesity need to be developed and then tested through research.
- *Measurement.* What are valid behavioral and environmental instruments for measuring progress (including intermediate outcomes) in obesity prevention in both the AI/AN target group and the general population?
- *Participatory Research.* What are creative ways that research designs can involve the AI/AN community in community assessments of the environment and other systems, consensus building, and participatory research?
- *Multi-site trials.* Multi-site research trials focusing on AI/ANs are needed so findings can be more generalizable.

Clinical Interventions

- *Maintenance of Weight Loss.* Can weight loss once achieved be maintained over time in the at-risk AI/AN population, and if so, what strategies are effective?
- *Drop-out Rates.* Drop-out rates are high in some AI/AN obesity treatment and prevention programs. What strategies are effective in sustaining adherence to intervention programs?
- *Barriers to Program Participation.* How can intervention programs successfully address constraints to program participation among AI/ANs (e.g., child care, transportation, social support, alcohol problems, and other social factors)?
- *Targeting At-Risk Groups.* What AI/AN at-risk groups should be targeted for early intervention to prevent obesity (e.g., women with prepregnancy and gestational diabetes, high birth weight babies, obese pregnant women, and obese children)?
- *Primary Prevention Intervention Points.* When is the critical time to begin intervention in order to prevent obesity among AI/AN children? (Note: IHS is currently examining their data to explore this issue).

Community-based Interventions

- *Family-focused Interventions.* What family processes and behaviors contribute to obesity in AI/ANs? What are the key intervention points during a family's life cycle? How can family-focused interventions be designed, and how can the effectiveness these interventions best be measured in the general population as well as with AI/AN families?
- *Effective Approaches.* Studies have indicated that AI/AN youth and adults are increasingly aware of and concerned about overweight/obesity and that they understand that obesity is related to dietary behavior. What type of community-based approaches that reflect the culture and traditions of AI/ANs are effective; for example, home-based and/or group methods?
- *Mediating Variables.* Several community and school-based studies targeting AI/ANs have found that although there was no change in BMI over time, there were changes in knowledge, attitudes, behaviors, or policies (e.g., physical activity levels, change in dietary intake, reduced TV watching, greater weight-related knowledge, school nutrition policies, safe community walking paths, increased access to healthy foods). What are the key mediating variables or proximal outcomes that need to be addressed in community/school-based interventions with respect to this target population? How can positive results regarding these outcomes be built upon to foster additional research and progress toward obesity prevention?
- *Interventions with Urban Indians.* What types of intervention strategies are most effective for addressing obesity in urban Indians?
- *Macroenvironmental Interventions.* What type of interventions with the general population as well as AI/ANs have been or can be implemented with respect to the macroenvironment (e.g., access to healthful foods, opportunities for physical activity, food advertising), and how effective have these interventions been?

REFERENCES

Action, K. J., Burrows, N. R., Moore, K., Querec, L., Geiss, L. S., Engelgau, M. M. (2002). Trends in diabetes prevalence among American Indian and Alaska native children, adolescents, and young adults. *American Journal of Public Health*, *92*, 9, 1485-1490.

Alaska Native Health Board (ANHB)/Alaska Native Epidemiology Center (ANEC). (2004). Final Report on The Alaska Traditional Diet Survey. Available at: http://www.arctichealth.org/ANHB_Final%20Report%20on%20the%20Alaska%20Traditional% 20Diet%20Survey_March%202004%20(ATDP_final).pdf

Allen, P., Thompson, J., Wolfe, V., Wilson, N., Whyte, A., Perez, G. & Herman, C. F. (2006a)*Lessons learned from a diabetes primary prevention educational intervention study.* 16th Annual Art and Science of Health Promotion Conference 2006 by American Journal of Health Promotion, Las Vegas, NV, March 20-24, Poster presentation.

Allen, P., Thompson, J., Wolfe, V., Wilson, N., Whyte, A., Perez, g & Herman C. (2006b). *Changes in Healthy Eating and Physical Activity Patterns Among Urban Native American Women in a Primary Prevention Study.* Presentation at the American Public Health Association November 2006 Annual Meeting.

Alves, J. (1993). Reaching Native Americans. *Journal of Extension*, *31*, 1, Spring.

Arehart-Treichel, J. (2005). Depression Risk Lower Among Native Americans. *Psychiatric News*, *40*, 19, 29.

Ballew, C., et al. (1997). Intake of nutrients and food sources of nutrients among the Navajo; findings from the Navajo Health and Nutrition Survey, *The Journal of Nutrition*, 127(10 Suppl), 2085S-2093S.

Baranowski, T., Anderson, C. & Carmack, C. (1998). Mediating variable framework in physical activity interventions: how are we doing? How might we do better? *American Journal of Preventive Medicine*, *14*, 4, 266-297.

Baranowski. T., Lin, L. S., Wetter, D. W., Resnicow, K. & Davis, Hearn, M. (1997). Theory as mediating variables: why aren't community interventions working as desired: *Annals of Epidemiology*, 7(suppl), S89-S95.

Barnes, P. M., Adams, P. F. & Powell-Griner E. (2005). Health Characteristics of the American Indian and Alaska Native Adult Population: United States, 1999-2003. *Advance Data from Vital and Health Statistics*, *356*.

Blackett, P. R., Taylor, T., Russell, D., Lu, M., Fesmire, J. & Lee, E. T. (1996). Lipoprotein changes in relation to body mass index in Native American adolescents. *Pediatric Research*, *40*, 77-81.

Bliss, R. (2004). Breaking Barriers to American Indian Nutrition Research. *Agricultural Research*, *52*, 7, 18-19

Boyer et al. (2005). Building a Community-Based Participatory Research Center to Investigate Obesity and Diabetes in Alaska Natives. *International Journal of Circumpolar Health*, *64*(3), 281-290.

Brave Heart M. (1998). The return to the sacred path: Healing the historical trauma and historical unresolved grief response among the Lakota. *Smith College Studies in Social Work*, *68*(3), 287-305.

Brave Heart, M. & DeBruyn, L. M. (1998). The American Indian Holocaust: Healing historical unresolved solved grief. *American Indian and Alaska Native Mental Health Research*, *8*, 60-82.

Broussard, B., Sugarman, J., Bachman-Carter, K., Booth, K., Stephenson, L. Strauss, K. & Gohdes, D. (1995). Toward Comprehensive Obesity Prevention Programs in Native American Communities. *Obesity Research*, 3 (suppl.2), 289S-297S.

Broussard, B., Sugarman, J., Bachman-Carter, K., Booth, K., Stephenson, L. Strauss, K. & Gohdes, D. (1995). Toward Comprehensive Obesity Prevention Programs in Native American Communities. *Obesity Research*, *3* (suppl.2), 289S-297S.

Broussard, B., Sugarman, J., Bachman-Carter, K., Booth, K., Stephenson, L., Strauss, K. & Gohdes, D. (1995). Toward Comprehensive Obesity Prevention Programs in Native American Communities. *Obesity Research*, *3*, 2, 289s-292s.

Broussard, B., Sugarman, J., Bachman-Carter, K., Booth, K., Stephenson, L. Strauss, K. & Gohdes, D. (1995). Toward Comprehensive Obesity Prevention Programs in Native American Communities. *Obesity Research*, *3* (suppl.2), 289S-297S.

Brown, A. & Brenton, B. (1994). Dietary survey of Hopi Native American elementary students. *Journal of the American Dietetic Association*, *94*, 517-522.

Burrows, N. R., Geiss, L. S., Engelgau, M. M. & Acton, K. J. (2000). Prevalence of diabetes among Native Americans and Alaska Natives, 1990-1997: An increasing burden. *Diabetes Care*, *23*, 1786-1790.

Caballero, B. Clay, T., Davis, S. M., Ethelbah, B., Holy Rock, B., Lohman, T., Norman, J., Story, M., Stone, E. J., Stephenson, L. & Stevens, J. (2003). Pathways: a school-based, randomized controlled trial for the prevention of obesity in American Indian schoolchildren. *American Journal of Clinical Nutrition*, *78*, 1030-1038.

Caballero, B., Himes, J., Lohman, T., Davis, S., Stevens, J., Evans, M., Going, S. & Pablo, J. (2003). *American Journal of Clinical Nutrition*, 78, 308-12.

Campos-Outcalt, D., Ellis, J., Aickin, M., Valencia, J., Wunsch, M. & Steele, L. (1995). Prevalence of Cardiovascular Disease Risk Factors in a Southwestern Native American Tribe. *Public Health Reports, 110.*

Casper, M., Rith-Najarian, S., Croft, J., Giles, W. & Donehoo, R. (1996). Blood Pressure, Diabetes, and Body Mass Index among Chippewa and Menominee Indians: The Inter-Tribal Heart Project Preliminary Data. *Public Health Reports*, *111*.

CDC. (2004). *American Indian and Alaska Native Community Partnership Guide: Supplement and Activity Plans.* Atlanta Georgia: U.S. Department of Health and Human Services, Public Health Service, Centers for Disease Control and Prevention, National Center for Chronic Disease Prevention and Health Promotion. Available at: http://ndep.nih.gov

CDC. (2005). Pediatric Nutrition Surveillance System (PedNSS). See: http://www.cdc.gov/pedness/what_is/pednss/.

Charles-Azure, J. & Little, E. (2005). Promotion of Healthier Beverages in Indian Communities. *The IHS Primary Care Provider*, *30*, 6.

Cole, N. (2002). *The Characteristics of Native American WIC Participants, On and Off Reservations*. Nutrition Assistance Program Report Series. May 2002. Report No. WIC-02- NAM. Alexandria VA: Office of Analysis, Nutrition and Evaluation, Food and Nutrition Service, USDA.

Cole, N. (2002). *The Characteristics of Native American WIC Participants, On and Off Reservations*. Alexandria, VA: U.S. Department of Agriculture, Food and Nutrition Service, Office of Analysis, Nutrition and Evaluation.

Conner, W. E., et al. (1978). The plasma lipids, lipoproteins, and diet of the Tarahumara Indians of Mexico. *American Journal of Clinical Nutrition*, *31*, 1131-1142.

Cullen, T. (2005). Personal Communication pertaining to data from IHS' Resource and Patient Management System (RPMS) data.

Cullen, T. (2005). Personal communication. Director, Office of Information Technology, IHS, 12300 Twinbrook Parkway, Suite 300, Rockville, Maryland 20852.

Cullen, T. (2006). Personal Communication. Director, Office of Information Technology, Indian Health Service, 12300 Twinbrook Parkway, Suite 300, Rockville, Maryland 20852.

Dabelea, D., Hanson, R. L., Bennett, P. H., Roumain, J., Knowler, W. C. & Pettitt, D. J. (1998). Increasing prevalence of Type II diabetes in American Indian children. *Diabetologia*, *41*, 8, 904-910.

Daniels, S. (2006). The Consequences of Childhood Overweight and Obesity. *The Future of Children*, *16*, 1, 47-67.

Davis, S. M. & Lambert, L. C. (2000). Body image and weight concerns among Southwestern American Indian preadolescent schoolchildren. *Ethnicity and Disease*, *10*, 2, 184-194

Davis, S. M., Lambert, L. C., Gomez, Y. & Skipper, B. (1995). Southwest Cardiovascular Curriculum Project: Study Findings for American Indian Elementary Students. *Journal of Health Education*, Supplement, *26*, 2: S-72 to S-81.

Davis, S., Clay, T., Smyth, M., Gitttelsohn, J., Arviso, V., Flint-Wagner, H., Holy Rock, B., Brice, R.A., Metcalfe, L., Stewart, D., Vu, M. & Stone, E. (2003). Pathways curriculum and family interventions to promote healthful eating and physical activity in American Indian schoolchildren. *Preventive Medicine*, *37*, S24-S34.

Davis, S., Gomez, Y., Lambert, L., & Skipper, B. (1993). Primary prevention of obesity in American Indian children. *Ann N Y Acad Sci*, *699*, 167-80.

De Cora, Loreli. (2006). Personal Communication. ldecora@seva.org

deGonzague, B., Receveur, O., Wedll, D. & Kuhnlein, H. (1999). Dietary intake and body mass index of adults in 2 Ojibwe communities. *Journal of the American Dietetic Association*, *99*, 6, 710-716.

Denny, C., Holtzmann, D. & Cobb, N. (2003). Surveillance for Health Behaviors of American Indians and Alaska Natives: Findings from the Behavioral Risk Factor Surveillance System, 1997-2000. *Morbidity & Mortality Weekly Report*, *52*, No. SS-7.

DHHS. (2001). *The Surgeon General's Call to Action To Prevent and Decrease Overweight and Obesity 2001*. Rockville, Maryland: U.S. Department of Health and Human Services, Public Health Service, Office of the Surgeon General.

DHHS. (2001a). The Surgeon General's Call to Action to Prevent and Decrease Overweight and *Obesity*. Rockville, Maryland: DHHS, Public Health Service, Office of the Surgeon General.

DHHS. (2001b). *Fact Sheet: Overweight and Obesity: At a Glance*. See http://www.surgeongeneral.gov/topics/obesity/calltoaction/fact_glance. htm

Diabetes Prevention Program (DPP) Research Group. (2002). The Diabetes Prevention Program (DPP). Description of lifestyle intervention. *Diabetes Care*, 25, 12: 2165-2171. Herman, C. 2006. Personal communication with Carla Herman, MD, MPH, Principal Investigator of Sharing Wisdom

Study, Professor of Medicine, Department of Internal Medicine, University of New Mexico, Center on Aging, Albuquerque, New Mexico.

Diabetes Prevention Program Research Group. (2000a). Reduction In The Incidence of Type 2 diabetes With Lifestyle Intervention or Metformin. *The New England Journal of Medicine*, *346*, 6, 393-403.

Diabetes Prevention Program Research Group. (2000b). The Diabetes Prevention Program (DPP). *Diabetes Care*, *25*, 12, 2165-2171.

Dietz, W. (1998). Health Consequences of Obesity in Youth: Childhood Predictors of Adult Disease. *Pediatrics*, *101*, 3, 518-525.

Dillinger, T., Jett, S., Macri, M. & Grivetti, L. (1999). Feast or famine? Supplemental food programs and their impact on two American Indian communities in California. *International Journal of Food Sciences and Nutrition*, *50*, 173-187.

Eisenberg, M. E., Neumark-Sztainer, D. & Story, M. (2003). Associations of Weight-Based Teasing and Emotional Well-Being among Adolescents. *Archives of Pediatrics and Adolescent Medicine*, *157*, 733-738.

Eisenman, J. C., Katzmarzyk, D. A., Arnall, V., Kanuho, C., Interpreter, C. & Malina, R. M. (2000). Growth and overweight of Navajo youth secular changes from 1955-1997. *International Journal of Obesity*, *24*, 211-218.

Eisenmann, J. C., Arnall, D., Kanuho, V., McArel, H. Growth Status & Obesity of Hopi Children. (2003). *American Journal of Human Biology*, *15*, 741-745.

Esparza, J., Fox, C., Harper, I. T., Bennett, P. H., Schulz, I. O., Valencia, M. E. & Ravussin, E. (2000). Daily energy expenditure in Mexican and USA Pima Indians: low physical activity as a possible cause of obesity. *International Journal of Obesity*, *24*, 55-59.

Fagot-Campagna, A., Pettit, D. J., Engelgau, M. M., Rios Burrows, N., Geiss, L. S. & Valdez, R. (2000). Type 2 diabetes among North American children and adolescents: an epidemiologic review and a public health perspective. *Journal of Pediatrics*, *136*, 664-672.

Finegold, K., Pindus, N., Wherry, L., Nelson, S., Triplett, T. & Capps, R. (2005). *Background Report on the Use and Impact of Food Assistance Programs on Indian Reservations.* Washington D.C. United States Department of Agriculture. Available at http://www.ers.usda.gov/Publications/CCR4/

Finegold, K., Pindus, N., Wherry, L., Nelson, S., Triplett, T. & Capps, R. (2005). *Background Report on the Use and Impact of Food Assistance Programs on Indian Reservations.* Washington D.C. United States

Department of Agriculture. Available at http://www.ers.usda.gov/Publications/CCR4/

Finkelstein, E., Khavjou, O., Mobley, L., Haney, D. & Will. J. (2004). Racial/Ethnic Disparities in Coronary Heart Disease Risk Factors among WISEWOMAN Enrollees. *Journal of Women's Health, 13*, 5, 503-518.

Fontvieille, A. M., Kriska, A. & Ravussin, E. (1993). Decreased physical activity in Pima Indian compared with Caucasian children. *International Journal of Obesity, 17*, 445-452.

Fontvielle, A. M., Kriska, A. & Ravussin, E. (1993). Decreased physical activity in Pima Indians compared with Caucasian children. *International Journal of Obesity Related Metabolic Disorders, 17*(8), 445-52.

Fox, M., Crepinsek, P., Connor, P. & Battaglia, M. (2001). School Nutrition Dietary Assessment Study – II. Summary of Findings. Alexandria VA: U.S. Department of Agriculture, Food and Nutrition Service, Office of Analysis, Nutrition and Evaluation.

Fox, M., Hamilton, W. & Biing-Hwan, L. (2004). *Effects of Food Assistance and Nutrition Programs on Nutrition and Health: Volume III, Literature Review*. Food and Nutrition Research Report No. 19-3. Washington D.C.: U.S. Department of Agriculture, Economic Research Service.

Freedman, D. C., Serdula, M. K., Percy, C. A., Ballew, C. & White, L. (1997). Obesity levels of lipids and glucose, and smoking among Navajo adolescents. *Journal of Nutrition, 127*(suppl), 21, 20S-27S.

Gallaher, M. M., Hauck, M. D., Yang-Oshida, M. & Serdula, M. K. (1991). Obesity among Mescalero Preschool Children. *American Journal of Diseases of Children, 145*(11), 1262-1265.

Ghodes, D. (1995). Diabetes in North American Indians and Alaska Natives. In: Group NDD (Ed), *Diabetes in America* (95-1468). Washington DC: National Institutes of Health, Publication, 95-1468.

Gilbert, T. J., Percy, C. A., Sugarman, J. R., Benson, L. & Percy, C. (1992). Obesity among Navajo adolescents. 1992. Relationship to dietary intake and blood pressure. *American Journal of Diseases of Children, 146*, 289-295.

Gittelsohn, J., Davis, S., Steckler, A., Ethelbah, B., Clay, T., Metcalfe, L. & Holy Rock, B. (2003). Pathways: lessons learned and future directions for school-based interventions among American Indians. *Preventive Medicine*; *37*, S107-S112.

Giuliano, A., Papenfuss, M., Guernsey De Zapien, J., Tilousi, S. & Nuvayestewa, L. (1998). Prevalence of Chronic Disease Risk and

Protective Behaviors among American Indian Women Living on the Hopi Reservation. *Annals of Epidemiology*, *8*(3), 160-167.

Giuliano, A., Papenfuss, M., Guernsey De Zapien, J., Tilousi, S. & Nuvayestewa, L. (1998). Prevalence of Chronic Disease Risk and Protective Behaviors among American Indian Women Living on the Hopi Reservation. *Annals of Epidemiology*, *8*(3), 160-167.

Goran, M. I., Kaskoun, M. C., Martinez, C., Kelly, B., Carpenter, W. H. & Hood, V. L. (1995). Energy expenditure and body fat distribution in Mohawk Indian children. *Pediatrics*, *95*, 89-95.

Gortmaker, S. L., Peterson, K., Wiecha, J., et al. (1999). Reducing obesity via a school-based interdisciplinary intervention among youth: Planet Health. *Archives of Pediatric Adolescent Medicine*, *153*, 409-418

Grant, R., Arcand, M., Plumage, C., White, M. & Fort Belknap College. (2000). Federal Food Programs, Traditional Foods and the Gros Ventre & Assiniboine Nations of the Fort Belknap Indian Reservation. See: http://www.nptao.arizona.edu/.

Gray, A. & Smith, C. (2003). Fitness, dietary intake, and body mass index in urban Native American youth. *Journal of the American Dietetic Association*, *103*, 9, 1187-1191.

Gray, R. S., Fabsitz, R. R., Cowan, L. D., Lee, E. T., Welty, T. K., Jablonski, K. A. & Howard, B. V. (2000). Relation of generalized and central obesity to cardiovascular risk factors and prevalent coronary heart disease in a sample of American Indians: the Strong Heart Study. *International Journal of Obesity*, *24*, 849-860.

Gray, S. & Smith, C. (2003). Fitness, dietary intake, and body mass index in urban Native American youth. *Journal of the American Dietetic Association*, *103*(9), 1187-1191.

Hall, T. R., Hickey, M. E. & Young, T. B. (1992). Evidence for recent increases in obesity and non- insulin-dependent diabetes mellitus in a Navajo community. *American Journal of Human Biology*, *4*, 547-553.

Harnack, L., Story, M. & Holy Rock, B. (1999). Diet and physical activity patterns of Lakota Indian adults. *Journal of the American Dietetic Association*, *99*(7), 829-835.

Harnack, L., Story, M., Holy Rock, B., Neumark-Sztainer, D., Jeffery, R. & French S. (1999). Nutrition Beliefs and Weight Loss Practices of Lakota Indian Adults. *Journal of Nutrition Education*; *31*, 1, 10-15.

Harrison, G. & Ritenbaugh, C. (1992). Obesity Among North American Indians. In: P. Bjorntorp & B Brodoff (Eds), *Obesity* (pp 610-618). Philadelphia: J.B. Lippincott Company.

Harvey-Bereno, J., Wellman, Al, Hood, V., Rourke, J. & Secker-Walker, R. (2000). Preventing obesity in American Indian children: When to begin. *Journal of the American dietetic Association*, *100*(5), Research, 5.

Harvey-Berino, J. & Rourke, J. (2003). Obesity Prevention on Preschool Native American Children: A Pilot Study Using Home Visiting. *Obesity Research*, *11*, 5, 606-611.

Harwell, T. S., Gohdes, D., Moore, K., McDowall, J. M., Smilie, J. G. & Helgerson, S. D. (2001). Cardiovascular Disease and Risk Factors in Montana American Indians and Non-Indians. *American Journal of Preventive Medicine*, *20*(3), 196-201.

Hasin, D., Goodwin, R., Stinson, F. & Grant, B. (2005). Epidemiology of Major Depressive Disorder. *Archives of General Psychiatry*, *62*, 1097-1106.

Hassel, C. (2006). Woodlands Wisdom: A Nutrition Program Interfacing Indigenous and Biomedical Epistemologies. *Journal of Nutrition, Education and Behavior*, *38*,114-120.

Heath, G., Wilson, R., Smith, J. & Leonard, B. (1991). Community-based exercise and weight control: diabetes risk reduction and glycemic control in Zuni Indians. *American Journal of Clinical Nutrition*, *53*, 1642S-1646S.

Hedley, A. A., Ogden, C. L., Johnson, C. L., Carroll, M. D., Curtin, L. R. & Flegal, K. M. (2004). Prevalence of Overweight and Obesity among US Children, Adolescents, and Adults, 1999-2002. *Journal of the American Medical Association*, *291*(23), 2847-2850.

Hillabrant, W., Rhoades, M., Pindus, N. & Trutko, J. (2001). *The Evaluation of the Tribal Welfare-to-Work Grants Program: Initial Implementation Findings*. Princeton, New Jersey: Mathematic Policy Research, Inc.

Hiwalker, R., Davis, J., Ward, C., Youngstrom, C., Li, W. & Feinauer E. (2002). The Relationship of Food Assistance Program Participation to Nutritional and Health Status, Diabetes Risk and Food Security Among the Northern Cheyenne. Unpublished report prepared for the U.S. Department of Agriculture, Washington D.C.

Hodge, F. (2007). *Final Report of the Diabetes Wellness Evidence-Based Project*. Atlanta, Georgia: Centers for Disease Control and Prevention.

Hodge, F. S., Pasqua A., Marquez, C. A. & Geishirt-Cantrell B. (2002). Utilizing traditional storytelling to promote wellness in American Indian communities. *Journal of Transcultural Nursing.*, *13*, 1, 6-11.

Hood, V. L., Kelly, B., Martinez, C., Shuman, S. & Secker-Walker, R. (1997). A Native American Community Initiative to Prevent Diabetes. *Ethnicity and Health*, *2*, 4, 277-285.

Hood,, V. L., Kelly, B., Martinez, C., Shuman, S. & Secker-Walker, R. (1997). A Native American Community Initiative to Prevent Diabetes. *Ethnicity and Health*, *2*, 4, 277-285.

Howard, B. F., Lee, E. T., Cowan, L. D., et al. (1995). Coronary heart disease prevalence and its relation to risk factors in American Indians. The Strong Heart Study. *American Journal of Epidemiology*, *142*, 254-268.

Hrdlicka, A. (1908). Psysiological and medical observations among the Indians of Southwestern United States and Northern Mexico. Washington D.C.: Smithsonian Institution, Bureau of Indian Ethnology Bulletin 34.

IHS (2004). Interim Report to Congress. Special Diabetes Program for Indians. Available at: www.ihs.gov/Medical/Programs/Diabetes/resources/r_rtc2004index.asp

IHS. (2001). IHS Report to Congress: Obesity Prevention and Control for American Indians and *Alaska Natives.* See: http://www.ihs.gov/hpdp/documents/obesitypreventionreport.doc

IHS. (2001). IHS Report to Congress: Obesity Prevention and Control for American Indians and *Alaska Natives.* See: http://www.ihs.gov/hpdp/documents/obesitypreventionreport.doc

IHS. (2005a). Healthy Children, Healthy Families, and Healthy Communities Initiative. Indian Health Service Head Start Program Final Report 2005. Contact Cheryl Wilson, IHS, Albuquerque New Mexico.

IHS. (2005b). 12-Area Summary Report Indian Health Service, Government Performance Results *Act*, *2005*. Rockville, Maryland: Indian Health Service

Indian Health Service (IHS), (2006). Facts on Indian Health Disparities. Rockville Marland: IHS. Kumanyika S. 1995. Obesity in Minority Populations. In K. Brownell & C. Fairburn (Eds), Eating Disorders and Obesity, A Comprehensive Handbook (431-437). New York: The Guilford Press.

Indian Health Service (IHS). (2001). IHS Report to Congress: Obesity Prevention and Control for American Indians and Alaska Natives. Available at: http://www.ihs.gov/hpdp/documents/obesitypreventionreport.doc.

Indian Health Service (IHS). (2001). *IHS Report to Congress: Obesity Prevention and Control for American Indians and Alaska Natives.*

Available at: http://www.ihs.gov/hpdp/documents/obesityprevention-report.doc

Indian Health Service (IHS). (2001). IHS Report to Congress: Obesity Prevention and Control for American Indians and Alaska Natives. Available at: http://www.ihs.gov/hpdp/documents/ obesityprevention-report.doc

Indian Health Service (IHS). (2006). *Indian Health Diabetes Best Practices: Community Advocacy and Diabetes*. Albuquerque, New Mexico: IHS, Division of Diabetes Treatment and Prevention. Available at: www.ihs.gov/medicalprograms/diabetes

Jackson, M. (1993). Height, weight and body mass index of American Indian school children, 1990-1991. *Journal of the American Dietetic Association, 93*, 10, 1136-1140.

Kileen, Martin. (2006). IHS, Albuquerque, New Mexico. Personal Communication. martin.kileen@ihs.hhs.gov.

Knowler, W. C., Pettitt, D. J., Saad, M. F. & Charles, M. A. (1991). Obesity in the Pima Indians: its magnitude and relationship with diabetes. *American Journal of Clinical Nutrition, 53*, 15435-15515.

Knowler, W. C., Pettitt, D. J., Saad, M. F. et al. (1991). Obesity in the Pima Indians: its magnitude and relationship with diabetes. *American Journal of Clinical Nutrition, 53*, 1543S-1551S.

Knowler, W. C., Pettitt, D. J., Saad, M. R. et al. (1991). Obesity in the Pima Indians: its magnitude and relationship with diabetes. *American Journal of Clinical Nutrition, 53*, 1543S-1551S.

Knowler, W.C. Pettitt, D., Mohammed, S., & Bennett, P. (1990). Diabetes Mellitus in the Pima Indians: Incidence, Risk Factors and Pathogenesis. *Diabetes/Metabolism Reviews, 6*, 1, 1-27.

Knowler, W.C., Pettitt, D.J., Savage, P.J., and Bennett, P.H. (1981). Diabetes incidence in Pima Indians: contributions of obesity and parental diabetes. *American Journal of Epidemiology, 113*, 144-156.

Koplan, J., Liverman, C. & Kraak, V. (2005). Preventing Childhood Obesity. Health in the Balance. p. 1. Washington D.C.: The National Academies Press.

Kriska, A., Saremi, A., Hanson, R., Bennett, P., Kobes, S., Willians, D. & Knowler, W. C. (2003). Physical Activity, Obesity, and the Incidence of Type 2 Diabetes in a High-Risk Population. *American Journal of Epidemiology. 158*, 7, 669-675.

Kumanyika, S. & Grier, S. (2006). Targeting Interventions for Ethnic Minority and Low-Income Populations. *The Future of Children, 16*, 1, 187-207.

Lee, E. T., Howard, B. V., Savage, P. J. et al. (1995). Diabetes and impaired glucose tolerance in three American Indian populations aged 45-74 years: The Strong Heart Study. *Diabetes Care*, *18*, 599-610

Liao, Y., Tucker, P. & Giles, W. H. (2003). Health Status of American Indians Compared with Other Racial/Ethnic Minority Populations – Selected States, 2001-2002. *Morbidity and Mortality Weekly Report*, *52*, 47, 1148.

Lindsay, R. S., Cook, V., Hanson, R. L., Salbe, A. D., Tataranni, A. & Knowler, D. C. (2002). Early excess weight gain of children in the Pima Indian population. *Pediatrics*, *109*(2), E33.

Luepker, R., Perry, C., McKinlay, S., et al. (1996). Outcomes of a field trial to improve children's dietary patterns and physical activity: The Child and Adolescent Trial for Cardiovascular Health. CATCH Collaborative Group. *JAMA*, *275*, 768-776.

Mahal, Z., Leach, R. & Jossefides, M. (2006). *Pediatric Height and Weight Study in American Indian and Alaska Native Population, 2001-2004. Final Report.* Rockville, Maryland: U.S. Department of Health and Human Services, Indian Health Service.

Manson, S., Beals, J., Klein, S., Croy, C. & AI-SUPERPFP Team. (2005). Social Epidemiology of Trauma Among 2 American Indian Reservation Populations. *American Journal of Public Health*, *95*, 5.

Marlow, E., Melkkus, G. D. & Bosma, A. M. (1998). STOP Diabetes! An Educational Model for Native American Adolescents in the Prevention of Diabetes. *The Diabetes Educator*, *24*, 4, 441-450.

McGinnis, J. M. & Foege, W. H. (1993). Actual causes of death in the United States. *Journal of the American Medical Association*, *270*, 2207-2212.

McGinnis, M. (2004). Obesity: An American Public Health Epidemic. *Expert Voices*, Issue 6, December 2004. NIHCM Foundation publication.

Mendlein, J. M., Freedman, D. S., Peter, D. G., Allen, B., Percy, C. A., Ballew, C., Mokdad, A. H. & White, L. L. (1997). Risk factors for coronary heart disease among Navajo Indians. *Journal of Nutrition*, *127*, 10S, 2099S.

Michel, K. L. (2004). The New Focus on Native American Cooking. *The Washington Post*, September, *22*, 2004.

Miller, P. (1994). *The Food Distribution Program on Montana's Indian Reservations.* Helena, MT: The Montana Department of Social and Rehabilitation Services and The Montana Hunger Coalition. Spring.

Moum, K. R., Holzman, G. S., Harwell, T., Parsons, S. L., Adams, S. D., Oser, C. S., Spense, M. R., Helgerson, S. D. & Gohdes, D. (2004). Increasing Rate of Diabetes in Pregnancy Among American Indian and White

Mothers in Montana and North Dakota, 1989-2000. *Maternal and Child Health Journal*, *8*(2).

Murphy, S. R. N. Breastfeeding Promotion Specialist, Diabetes Center of Excellence, Phoenix Indian Medical Center. 4212 North 16th Street, Phoenix, AZ 85016. Suzan.Murphy@his.gov. Personal communication about unpublished study.

Must A. & Strauss, R. S. (1999). Risks and consequences of childhood and adolescent obesity. *International Journal of Obesity Related Metabolic Disorders*, 1999, *23*(suppl): S2-S11.

Nader, P. R., Stone, E. J., Lytle, L. A., et al. (1999). Three-year maintenance of improved diet and physical activity: the CATCH cohort. *Archives of Pediatric Adolescent Medicine*, *153*, 695-704.

Narayan, K. M., Venkat, Hoskin, M., Kozak, D., Kriska, A. M., Hanson, R. I., Pettit, D. J., Nagi, D. K., Bennett, P. H. & Knowler, W. C. (1998). Randomized Clinical Trial of Lifestyle Interventions in Pima Indians: a Pilot Study. *Diabetic Medicine*, *15*, 66-72.

National Diabetes Education Program (NDEP). *Changing the Way Diabetes is Treated: An Update on Outreach and Progress. The National Diabetes Education Program 1997-2003.* Bethesda, Maryland: U.S. Department of Health and Human Services, NIDDK, CDC, NDEP.

National Institutes of Health (NIH) (2004). *Strategic Plan for NIH Obesity Research. A Report of the NIH Obesity Research Task Force.* Bethesda, Maryland: U.S. Department of Health and Human Services, NIH, Publication No. 04-5493.

National Research Council Committee on Diet and Health (NRCCDH). 1989. *Diet and Health: Implications for Reducing Chronic Disease.* Washington DC: National Academy Press.

National Research Council Committee on Diet and Health (NRCCDH). (1989). *Diet and Health: Implications for Reducing Chronic Disease.* Washington DC: National Academy Press.

Neel, J. V. (1962). Diabetes mellitus: a "thrifty" genotype rendered detrimental by progress? *American Journal of Human Genetics*, *14*, 353-362.

Neumark-Sztainer, D., Story, M., Resnick, M. & Blum R. (1997). Psychosocial concerns and weight control behaviors among overweight and nonoverweight Native American adolescents. *Journal of the American Dietetic Association*, *97*, 6, 598-604.

Neumark-Sztainer, D., Story, M., Resnick, M. & Blum, R. (1997). Psychosocial concerns and weight control behaviors among overweight and nonoverweight Native American adolescents. *Journal of the American Dietetic Association*, *97*, 6, 598-604.

North, K. E., MacCluer, J. W., Williams, J. T., Welty, T. K., Best, L. G., Lee, E. T., Fabsitz, R. R. & Howard, B. V. (2003). Evidence for distinct genetic effects on obesity and lipid-related CVD risk factors in diabetic compared to nondiabetic American Indians: the Strong Heart Family Study. *Diabetes Metabolism Research and Reviews*, *19*, 140-147.

Ogden, C. L., Flegal, K.M., Carroll, M. D. & Johnson, C. L. (2002). Prevalence and Trends in Overweight Among US Children and Adolescents, 1999-2000. *Journal of the American Medical Association*, 288 (14), 1728-1732,

Ogden, C., Carroll, M., Curtin, L., McDowell, M., Tabak, C. & Flegal, K. (2006). Prevalence of Overweight and Obesity in the United States, 1999-2004. *Journal of the American Medical Association*, *295*, 13.

Ogden, C., Flegal, K., Carroll, M. & Johnson, C. (2002). Prevalence and trends in overweight among US children and adolescents, 1999-2000. *Journal of the American Medical Association*, *288*, 14, 1728-1732.

ORC, Macro. (2003). *Move It! Campaign Evaluation Activities – Final Report.* Atlanta Georgia: National Diabetes Education Program, Division of Diabetes Translation, National Center for Chronic Disease Prevention and Health Promotion.

Paradis, G., Levesque, L., Macaulay, A. C., Cargo, M., McComber, A., Kirby, R., Receveur, O., Kishchuck, N. & Potvin, L. (2005). Impact of a Diabetes Prevention Program on Body Size, Physical Activity and Diet Among Kanienkeha:ka (Mohawk) Children 6 to 11 Years Old: 8-Year Results from the Kahnawake Schools Diabetes Prevention Project. *Pediatrics*, *115*, 2, 333-339.

Pareo-Tubbeh, S., Shorty, M., Bauer, M. & Agbolosoo, E. (2000). The Variety, Affordability, and Availability of Healthful Foods at Convenience Stores and Trading Posts on the Navajo Reservation. See: http://www. nptao.arizona.edu/

Pargee, D., Lara-Albers, E. & Puckett, K. (1999). Building on Tradition: Promoting Physical Activity with American Indian Community Coalitions. *Journal of Health Education*, *30*, 2, S-37-S-43.

Parrish, D. (2002). Nutrition Assessment and Education for Keweenaw Bay Ojibwa. Unpublished report. Washington D.C.: U.S. Department of Agriculture.

Paxon, C., Donahue, E., Orleans, T. & Grisso, J. A. (2006). Introducing the Issue. *The Future of Children*, *16*(1), 3-17.

Pettitt, D., Nelson, R., Saad, M., Bennett, P. & Knowler, W. (1993). Diabetes and Obesity in the Offspring of Pima Indian Women with Diabetes During Pregnancy. 1993. *Diabetes Care*, *16* (Supplement 1), January.

Phillips and Finn (2000). Dietary Choices and Weight Loss Practices Among Cheyenne River Lakota Households. See http://www.nptao.arizona.edu.

Phillips, J. & Finn, J. (2000). Dietary Choices and Weight Loss Practices Among Cheyenne River Lakota Households. See http://www.nptao.arizona.edu

Phillips, J. & Finn, J. (2000). Dietary Choices and Weight Loss Practices Among Cheyenne River Lakota Households. See http://www.nptao.arizona.edu

Pine, D. S. et al. (2001). The Association between Childhood Depression and Adulthood Body Mass Index. *Pediatrics*, *107*, 1049-1056.

Powell, L., Slater, S. & Chaloupka F. J. (2004). The relationship between community physical activity settings and race, ethnicity and socioeconomic status. *Evidence-Based Preventive Medicine*, *1*(2), 135-144.

Power, C., Lake, J. K. & Cole, T. J. (1997). Measurement and long term risks of child and adolescent fatness. *International Journal of Obesity*, *21*, 507-526.

PRC, (2006). Factsheet: American Indian and Alaska Native Heritage Month. Population Resource Center, 1725 K Street NW, Suite 1102, Washington DC 20006.

Ravussin, E. (1995). Metabolic Differences and the Development of Obesity. *Metabolism*, *44*(9), Suppl 3 (September), 12-14.

Reid, R. & Rhoades, E. (2000). Cultural Considerations in Providing Care to American Indians. In: E. Rhoades (Ed), *American Indian Health* (418-425). Baltimore: The Johns Hopkins University Press.

Rinderknecht, K. & Smith, C. (2002). Body image perceptions among urban Native American youth. *Obesity Research*, *10*, 315-327.

Risica, P. M., Ebbesson, S. O., Schraer, C. D., Nobmann, E. D. & Caballero, B. H. (2000). Body fat distribution in Alaskan Eskimos of the Bering Straits region: the Alaskan Siberia Project. *International Journal of Obesity*, *24*,171-179.

Rosso, R. & Faux, M. (2003). *Characteristics of Food Stamp Households: Fiscal Year 2002*. Alexandria, VA: U.S. Department of Agriculture, Food and Nutrition Service. Office of Analysis, Nutrition and Evaluation.

Roubideaux, Y., Moore, K., Avery, C., Muneta, B., Knight, M. & Buchwald, D. (2000). Diabetes Education Materials: Recommendations of Tribal

Leaders, Indian Health Professionals, and American Indian Community Members. *The Diabetes Educator*, *26*, 2, 290-294.

Salbe, A. D., Weyer, C. Lindsay, R. S., Ravussin, E., Tataranni, P. A. (2002). Assesing risk factors for obesity between childhood and adolescence: Birth weight, childhood adiposity, parental obesity, insulin and leptin. *Pediatrics*, 110(2Pt 1), 299-306.

Salbe, A. D., Weyer, C., Lindsay, R. S., Ravussin, E. & Tataranni, P. A. (2002). Assesing risk factors for obesity between childhood and adolescence: Birth weight, childhood adiposity, parental obesity, insulin and leptin. *Pediatrics*, *110*(2Pt 1), 299-306.

Satterfield, D., Volansky, M., Caspersen, C., Engelgau, M., Bowman, B., Gregg, E., Geiss, L., Hosey, G., May, J. & Vinicor, F. (2003). Community-Based Lifestyle Interventions to Prevent Type 2 Diabetes. *Diabetes Care*, *26*, 9, 2643-2652.

Seva Foundation. (2006). Diabetes Talking Circles Now a "Best Practice." New Recognition by Indian Health Service. Available at: http://www.seva.org/news015.php

Shanklin, D., Usher, C. & Wildfire, J. (1992). Nutrition Education Needs and Services Among American Indians Participating in a Federal Food Assistance Program. *Journal of Nutrition Education*, *24*, 6, 298-305.

Sherwood, N., Harnack. L. & Story, M. (2000). Weight-loss practices, nutrition beliefs, and weight- loss program preferences of urban American Indian women. *Journal of the American Dietetic Association*, *100*, 4, 442-446.

Signorielli, N. & Staples, J. (1997). Television and children's conceptions of nutrition. *Health Communication*, *9*, 281-301.

Smedley, B. D. & Syme, S. L. (2000). *Promoting health: intervention strategies from social and behavioral research.* Washington, DC. Institute of Medicine, National Academy Press.

Smith, C. & Rinderknecht, K. (2003). Obesity Correlates with Increased Blood pressures in Urban Native American Youth. American Journal of Human Biology 15, 78-90.

Smith, C. & Rinderknecht, K. (2003). Obesity correlates with increased blood pressures in urban Native American youth. *American Journal of Human Biology*, *25*, 78-90.

Smith, J. & Wiedman, D. (2000). Lessons in Basket Weaving and Traditional Wisdom: Partnering with Elders in Alaska Aleutian Communities Enhance Success of WIC. *Journal of Family and Consumer Sciences*, *92*, 2, 25-27.

Steckler, A., Ethelbah, B., Martin, C. J., Stewart, D., Pardilla, M., Gittelsohn, J., Stone, E., Fenn, D., Smyth , M. & Vu, M. (2003). Pathways process evaluation results: a school-based prevention trial to promote healthful diet and physical activity in American Indian third, fourth, and fifth grade students. *Preventive Medicine*, *37*, S80-90.

Steinman, E. (2005). Native Americans suffer from historical trauma, researcher says. *The United Methodist Church News*, July 27, 2005. http://www.umc.org/site/c.gjJTJbMUIuE/b.928147/k.CB36/Native_Americans_suffer_from_hist orical_trauma_researcher_says.htm.

Stettler, N., Zemel, B. S., Kumanyika, S. & Stallings, V. A. (2002). Infant weight gain and childhood overweight status in a multicenter cohort study. *Pediatrics*, *109*(2), 194-199.

Story, M., Evans, M., Fabsitz, R. R. Clay, T. E., Holy Rock, B. & Broussard, B. (1999). The epidemic of obesity in American Indian communities and the need for childhood obesity-prevention programs. 1999. *American Journal of Clinical Nutrition*, *69*, 747S-754S.

Story, M., Evans, M., Fabsitz, R. R., Clay, T. E., Holy Rock, B. & Broussard, B. (1999). The epidemic of obesity in American Indian communities and the need for childhood obesity- prevention programs. *American journal of Clinical Nutrition*, *69*(suppl), 747S-754S.

Story, M., Evans, M., Fabsitz, R. R., Clay, T., Holy Rock, B. & Broussard, B. (1999). The epidemic of obesity in American Indian communities and the need for childhood obesity- prevention programs. *American Journal of Clinical Nutrition*, *69*, (suppl), 747S-754S.

Story, M., French, S. A., Resnick, M. D. & Blum, R. W. (1995). Ethnic/racial and socioeconomic differences in dieting behaviors and body image perceptions in adolescents. *International Journal of Eating Disorders*, *18*, 2, 173-179.

Story, M., Hauck, F. R., Broussard, B. A., White, L. L., Resnick, M. D. & Blum, R. W. (1994). Weight perceptions and weight control practices in American Indian and Alaska Native Adolescents. A national survey. *Archives of Pediatric Adolescent Medicine*, *148*, 6, 567-571.

Story, M., Snyder, P., Anliker, J., Cunningham-Sabo, L., Weber, J., Ring, K., Platero, H. & Stone, E. (2002). Nutrient content of school meals in elementary schools on American Indian reservations. *Journal of the American Dietetic Association*, *102*, 2, 253.

Story, M., Stevens, J., Evans, M., Cornell, C., Juhaeri, Gittelsohn, J., Going, S., Clay, T. & Murray, D. (2001). Weight Loss Attempts and Attitudes toward Body Size, Eating, and Physical Activity in American Indian

Children: Relationship to Weight Status and Gender. *Obesity Research*, *9*, 356-363.

Story, M., Stevens, J., Himes, J., Stone, E., Holy Rock, B., Ethelbah, B. & Davis, S. (2003). Obesity in American-Indian children: prevalence, consequences, and prevention. *Preventive Medicine*, *37*, S3-S12.

Story, M., Stevens, J., Himes, J., Stone, E., Holy Rock, B., Ethelbah, B. & Davis, S. (2003). Obesity in American-Indian children: prevalence, consequences, and prevention. *Preventive Medicine*, *37*, S3-S12.

Story, M., Stevens, J., Himes, J., Stone, E., Holyrock, B., Ethelbah, B. & Davis, S. (2003). Obesity in American-Indian children: prevalence, consequences, and prevention. *Preventive Medicine*, *37*, S3-S12.

Story, M., Stevens, J., Himes, J., Stone, E., Holyrock, B., Ethelbah, B. & Davis, S. (2003). Obesity in American-Indian children: prevalence, consequences, and prevention. *Preventive Medicine*, *37*, S3-S12.

Story, M., Stevens, J., Himes, J., Stone, E., Holyrock, B., Ethelbah, B. & Davis, S. (2003). Obesity in American-Indian children: prevalence, consequences, and prevention. *Preventive Medicine*, *37*, S3-S12.

Story, M., Stevens, J., Himes, J., Stone, E., Holyrock, B., Ethelbah, B. & Davis, S. (2003). Obesity in American-Indian children: prevalence, consequences, and prevention. *Preventive Medicine*, *37*, S3-S12.

Story, M., Strauss, K., Gilbert, T. & Broussard, B. (2000). Nutritional Health and Diet-Related Conditions. In E.R.Rhoades (Ed), *American Indian Health: Innovations in Health Care, Promotion, and Policy* (201-220). Baltimore and London: The Johns Hopkins University Press.

Story, M., Strauss, K., Gilbert, T. & Broussard, B. (2004). Nutritional Health and Diet-Related Conditions. 2004. In E.R.Rhoades (Ed), *American Indian Health: Innovations in Health Care, Promotion, and Policy* (pp 201-220). Baltimore and London: The Johns Hopkins University Press.

Story, M., Strauss, K., Gilbert, T. J. & Broussard, B. A. (2000). Nutritional Health and Diet- Related Conditions. In E.R. Rhoades (Ed), *American Indian Health* (201-220). Baltimore and London: The Johns Hopkins University Press.

Story, M., Strauss, K., Zephier, E. & Broussard, B. (1998). Nutritional concerns in American Indian and Alaska Native children: Transitions and future directions. *Journal of the American Dietetic Association*, *98*, 2, 170-177.

Strauss, R. S. & Pollack, H. A. (2003). Social Marginalization of Overweight Children. *Archives of Pediatrics and Adolescent Medicine*, *157*, 746-752.

Struthers, R., Hodge, F. S., Geishirt-Cantrell, B. & De Cora, L. (2003a). Participant Experiences of Talking Circles on Type 2 Diabetes in Two Northern Plains American Indian Tribes. *Qualitative Health Research, 13*, 8, 1094-1115.

Struthers, R., Kaas, M., Hill, D. L., Hodge, F., DeCora, L. & Geishirt-Cantrell, B. (2003). Providing Culturally Appropriate Education on Type 2 Diabetes to Rural American Indians: Emotions and Racial Consciousness. *Journal of Rural Community Psychology*, E6, 1.

Sugarman, J. R., Gilbert, T. J., Percy, C. A. & Peter, D. G. (1992). Serum cholesterol concentrations among Navajo Indians. *Public Health Reports, 107*, 92-99.

Sugarman, J. R., Warren, C. W., Oge, L. & Helgerson, S. D. (1992). Using the behavioral risk factors surveillance system to monitor Year 2000 objectives among American Indians. *Public Health Reports*, 107, 449-456.

Sugarman, J. R., White, L. L. & Gilbert, T. J. (1990). Evidence for a secular change in obesity, height, and weight among Navajo Indian schoolchildren. *American Journal of Clinical Nutrition, 52*, 960-966,

Sugarman, J., Hickey, M., Hall, T. & Gohdes D. (1990). The changing epidemiology of diabetes mellitus among Navajo Indians. *Western Journal of Medicine, 153*, 140-145.

Swinburn, B. A., Nyomba, B. L., Saad, M. F., et al. (1991). Insulin resistance associated with lower rates of weight gain in Pima Indians. *Journal of Clinical Investigation, 88*, 168-173.

Teufel, N. & Dufour, D. (1990). Patterns of food use and nutrient intake of obese and non-obese Hualapai Indian women of Arizona. *Journal of the American Dietetic Association, 90*, 9, 1229-1235.

Teufel, N. & Ritenbaugh, C. (1998). Development of a Primary Prevention Program: Insight Gained in the Zuni Diabetes Prevention Program. *Clinical Pediatrics, 37*, 2, 131-141.

The Diabetes Prevention Program (DPP) Research Group. (2002). The Diabetes Prevention Program (DPP). *Diabetes Care, 25*, 12, 2165-2171.

The Diabetes Prevention Program Research Group. (2002). *Reduction in the Incidence of Type 2* Diabetes with Lifestyle Intervention or Metformin. *New England Journal of Medicine, 346*, 6, 393-403.

The Look AHEAD Research Group. (2003). Look AHEAD (Action for Health in Diabetes): Design and Methods for a Clinical trial of Weight Loss for the Prevention of Cardiovascular Disease in Type 2 Diabetes. *Controlled Clinical Trials, 24*, 610-628.

Thomas, S. L. & Cook, D. (2005). Breastfeeding Duration and Prevalence of Overweight Among 4-to 5-Year Olds. *The IHS Primary Care Provider*, *30*(4), April 2005.

Thompson, J. L., Davis, S. M., Gittelsohn, J., Going, S., Becenti, A., Metcalfe, L., Stone, E., Harnack, L. & Ring, K. (2001). Patterns of Physical Activity Among American Indian Children: An Assessment of Barriers and Support. *Journal of Community Health*, *26*(6), 423-445.

U. S. Department of Agriculture (USDA) (2004a). *Obesity, Poverty and Participation in Food Assistance Programs*, FSP-04-PO. Alexandria, VA: USDA, Office of Analysis, Nutrition and Evaluation, Food and Nutrition Office.

U. S. Department of Agriculture (USDA). (1990). *Evaluation of the Food Distribution Program on Indian Reservations. Vol 1, Final Report.* Washington D.C.: USDA, Food and Nutrition Service, Office of Analysis and Evaluation.

U. S. Department of Agriculture (USDA). (2005). Food Distribution Programs on Indian Reservations. Frequently Asked Questions. Available at: http://www.fns.usda.gov/fdd/faqs/fdpirfaq.htm.

U. S. Department of Agriculture (USDA). (2006). Annual State Level Data: Total WIC Program Participation, FY 1999-2003. Available at: http://www.fns.usda.gov/pd/wifypart.htm.

U. S. Department of Agriculture. (2004b). Food and Nutrition Service, FNS National Data Book. U. S. Department of Agriculture (USDA). 2004c. National Level Summary Table: Participation in the Indian Reservation and Commodity Supplemental Food Programs, and Meals Served in the Nutrition Services Incentive Program, FY 1969-2003. Available at: http://www.fns.usda.gov/pd/fdpart.htm.

U. S. Department of Health and Human Services (DHHS). (2001). *The Surgeon General's call to prevent and decrease overweight and obesity.* Rockville, MD: U.S. Department of Health and Human Services, Public Health Services, Office of the Surgeon General. Available from U.S. GPO, Washington.

U. S. Department of Health and Human Services (DHHS). (2005). *Trends in Indian Health 2000-2001*. Rockville MD: U.S. Department of Health and Human Services, Indian Health Service.

U. S. General Accounting Office, Food Assistance Programs. (1989). Report to Congress: Food Assistance Programs. Nutritional Adequacy of Primary Food Programs on Four Indian Reservations. Washington, D.C.: General Accounting Office.

U. S. News and World Report. 2005. Health spending soars for obesity. June 27, 2005.

U.S. Census Bureau. (2006). *We the People: American Indians and Alaska Natives in the United States. Census 2000 Special Reports.* Washington DC: U.S. Census Bureau, Economics and Statistics Administration, U.S. Department of Commerce.

U.S. Census. (2000). *We the People: American Indians and Alaska Natives in the United States.* See: http://www.census.gov/prod/2006pubs/censr-28.pdf.

U.S. Department of Agriculture (USDA), National Data Bank (NDB). Data from the NDB, Food and Nutrition Service (FNS), USDA. Obtained through personal communication with Nancy Theodore, FNS, FDPIR, USDA.

U.S. Department of Health and Human Services (DHHS). 2001. *The Surgeon General's Call to Action To Prevent and Decrease Overweight and Obesity.* Rockville, MD: DHHS, Public Health Service, Office of the Surgeon General.

U.S. Department of Health and Human Services (U.S. DHHS). (2001). *The Surgeon General's Call to Action To Prevent and Decrease Overweight and Obesity.* Rockville, Maryland: U.S. DHHS, Public Health Service, Office of the Surgeon General.

University of North Carolina at Chapel Hill. A New Leaf...Choices for Healthy Living. Chapel Hill, North Carolina: Center for Health Promotion and Disease Prevention.

Walston, J., Silver, K., Bogardus, C., et al. (1995). Time onset of non-insulin-dependent diabetes mellitus and genetic variation in the β3-adrenergic-receptor gene. *New England Journal of Medicine*, *333*, 343-347.

Walters, K. & Simoni, J. (2002). Reconceptualizing Native Woman's Health: An "Indigenist" Stress–Coping Model. *American Journal of Public Health*, *92*, 4, 520-524.

Washington Post. (2006). Health Experts Warn of Obesity Pandemic. September, 4.

Waters, K. & Simoni, J. (2002). Reconceptualizing Native Women's Health: An "Indigenist" Stress-Coping Model. *American Journal of Public Health*, *92*, 4, 524.

Weiss, K. M., Ferrell, R. E. & Hanis, C. L. (1984). A New World syndrome of metabolic diseases with a genetic and evolutionary basis. *Yearbook of Physical Anthropology*, *27*, 153.

Welty, T. (1991). Health Implications of Obesity in American Indians and Alaska Natives. *American Journal of Clinical Nutrition*, *53*, 1616S-20S.

Welty, T. (1991). Health implications of obesity in American Indians and Alaska Natives. *American Journal of Clinical Nutrition*, *53*, 1616S-20S.

Welty, T. K., Rhoades, D. A., Yeh, F., Lee, E. T., Cowan, L. D., Fabsitz, R. R., Robbins D. C., Devereux, R. B., Henderson, J. A. & Howard, B. (2002). Changes in Cardiovascular Disease Risk Factors among American Indians: The Strong Heart Study. *Annuals of Epidemiology*, *12*, 97-106.

Whitbeck, L., Adams, G., Hoyt, D. & Chen, X. (2004). Conceptualizing and Measuring Historical Trauma Among American Indian People. *American Journal of Community Psychology*, 33, Nos. ¾.

White, L. L., Ballew, C., Gilbert, T. J., Mendlein, J. M., Mokdad, A. H. & Strauss, K. F. (1997). Weight, body image, and weight control practices of Navajo Indians: findings from the Navajo Health & Nutrition survey. *Journal of Nutrition*, *127*, 2094S-2098S.

White, L. L., Ballew, C., Gilbert, T. J., Mendlein, J. M., Mokdad, A. H. & Strauss, K. F. Psychosocial and behavioral correlates of dieting and purging in Native American adolescents. *Pediatrics*, *99*, e8.

White, L., Ballew, C., Gilbert, T. J., Mendlein, J. M., Mokdad, A. H. & Strauss, K. F. (1997). Weight, body Image, and Weight control Practices of Navajo Indians: Findings from the Navajo Health and Nutrition Survey, *The Journal of Nutrition*, *127*, 10S, 2094S-2098S.

Willging C, Helitzer, D. & Thompson J. (2006). "Sharing Wisdom": Lessons learned during the development of a diabetes prevention intervention for urban American Indian women. *Evaluation and Program Planning*, in press.

Wilson, C., Cullen, T., Moore, K., Roubideaux, Y., Valdez, L., Vanderwagen, W. & Acton, K. (2005). Diabetes Outcomes in the Indian Health System During the Era of the Special Diabetes Program for Indians and the government Performance and Results Act. *American Journal of Public Health*, Vol *95*, No. 9: 1518-1522.

Wilson, P., O'Mears, S., Summerhall, C. & Kelley, S. (2003). The prevention and treatment of childhood obesity. *Quality and Safety in Health Care*, *12*, 65-74.

Witmer, J. M., Hensel, M. R., Holck, P. S., Ammerman, A. S. & Will, J. C. (2004). Heart Disease Prevention for Alaska Native Women: A Review of Pilot Findings. *Journal of Women's Health*, *13*, 5, 569-578.

Witmer, J., Hensel, M., Holck, P., Ammerman, A. & Will, J. (2004). Heart Disease Prevention for Alaska Native Women: A Review of Pilot Study Findings. *Journal of Women's Health, 13*, 5, 569-578.

Wright, A. (1993). Maternal Employment and Infant Feeding Practices among the Navajo. *Medical Anthropology Quarterly*, 7(3), 260-280.

Yurgalevitch, S. M., Kriska, A. M., Welty, T. K, Go, O., Robbins, D. C. & Howard, B. V. (1998). Physical activity and lipids and lipoproteins in American Indians ages 45-74. *Medical Science Sports Exercise, 30*(4), 543-549.

Zephier, E., Himes, J. H. & Story, M. (1999). Prevalence of overweight & obesity in American Indian school children and adolescents in the Aberdeen area: a population study. *International Journal of Obesity Related Metabolic Disorders, 23*(suppl), S28-30.

Zephier, E., Himes, J., Story, M. & Zhou, X. (2006). Increasing Prevalences of Overweight and Obesity in Northern Plains American Indian Children. *Archives of Pediatric Adolescent Medicine, 160*, 34-39.

Zurlo, F., Lillioja, S., Esposito-Del Puente, A., et al. (1990). Low ratio of fat to carbohydrate oxidate as predictor of weight gain: study of 24-h RQ. *American Journal of Physiology, 259*, E650-E657.

End Notes

[1] *Strong in Body and Spirit* is a five session curriculum that is designed to help people eat healthy foods and increase exercise and is targeted to Native American adults with diabetes. Funding for the original version was provided by NIDDK and developed by the U of New Mexico's Office of Native American Diabetes Programs (NADP). CDC's Native Diabetes Wellness Program funded NADP to update this resource. It has been disseminated to 94 tribes, was is important not to assume that all Native Americans practice their traditions to the same degree or that they share similar traditions. The intervention consisted of five sessions (2 hours each) held monthly for 5 months and led by community-based Native American health educators. These sessions addressed the topics of physical activity, eating more vegetables and less fat, reducing intake of sweetened beverages and processed high sugar foods, social support, and maintenance of healthy lifestyle behavior changes. The sessions included a few minutes of moderate or light physical activity, discussions of behavior changes over the past month, didactic lessons and discussion, and healthy behavior goal setting for the month ahead.

In: Obesity Among American Indians … ISBN: 978-1-63463-486-1
Editor: Taylor Plaskett

Chapter 2

PREVALENCE OF OBESITY AMONG ADULTS: UNITED STATES, 2011–2012*

Cynthia L. Ogden, Margaret D. Carroll, Brian K. Kit and Katherine M. Flegal

KEY FINDINGS

Data from the National Health and Nutrition Examination Survey, 2011–2012

- More than one-third (34.9%) of adults were obese in 2011–2012.
- In 2011–2012, the prevalence of obesity was higher among middle-aged adults (39.5%) than among younger (30.3%) or older (35.4%) adults.
- The overall prevalence of obesity did not differ between men and women in 2011–2012. Among non-Hispanic black adults, however, 56.6% of women were obese compared with 37.1% of men.
- In 2011–2012, the prevalence of obesity was higher among non-Hispanic black (47.8%), Hispanic (42.5%), and non-Hispanic white (32.6%) adults than among non-Hispanic Asian adults (10.8%).

* This is an edited, reformatted and augmented version of NCHS Data Brief, No. 131, issued by the National Center for Health Statistics, October 2013.

- The prevalence of obesity among adults did not change between 2009–2010 and 2011–2012.

The health risks associated with obesity [1] make reducing the high prevalence of obesity a public health priority [2]. Previous publications have shown both racial and ethnic disparities in obesity prevalence and no change in the prevalence of obesity among adults since 2003–2004 [3,4]. National obesity prevalence estimates for non-Hispanic Asian persons are possible for the first time, using newly available data. This report presents national estimates of obesity among adults in the United States in 2011–2012, based on measured weight and height.

Keywords: Obese adults, National Health and Nutrition Examination Survey

What Was the Prevalence of Obesity Among Adults in 2011–2012?

More than one-third (age-adjusted 34.9%, crude 35.1%) of U.S. adults were obese in 2011–2012. Overall, the prevalence of obesity among middle-aged adults aged 40–59 was higher than among younger adults aged 20–39 or older adults aged 60 and over (Figure 1).

Men aged 40–59 had a higher prevalence of obesity (39.4%) than did men aged 20–39 (29.0%) and men aged 60 and over (32.0%). However, there was no difference in the prevalence of obesity between men aged 20–39 and those aged 60 and over. Among women, the prevalence of obesity did not differ between those aged 40–59 and 60 and over (39.5% compared with 38.1%). The prevalence of obesity among younger women was lower than among either middle-aged or older women.

Were Differences Seen in the Prevalence of Obesity Among Adults by Race and Hispanic Origin in 2011–2012?

The prevalence of obesity among non-Hispanic Asian adults (10.8%) was lower than among non- Hispanic white (32.6%), Hispanic (42.5%), and non-Hispanic black (47.8%) adults (Figure 2). The prevalence of obesity among

Hispanic men (40.1%) was higher than among non-Hispanic Asian (10.0%) and non-Hispanic white (32.4%) men. The prevalence of obesity was higher among non-Hispanic black women (56.6%) than among Hispanic (44.4%), non-Hispanic white (32.8%), and non-Hispanic Asian (11.4%) women.

The only difference by sex was found among non-Hispanic black adults: 56.6% of non-Hispanic black women were obese compared with 37.1% of non-Hispanic black men.

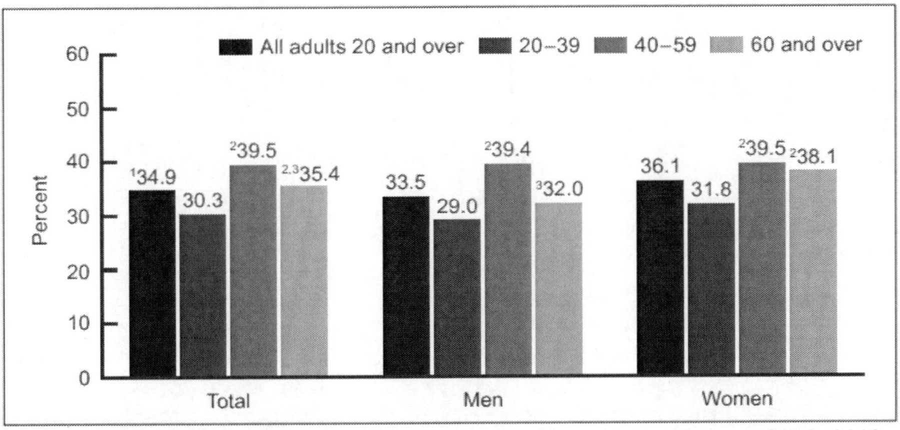

Source: CDC/NCHS, National Health and Nutrition Examination Survey, 2011–2012.

Note: Estimates are age-adjusted for all adults aged 20 and over by the direct method to the 2000 U.S. census population using the age groups 20–39, 40–59, and 60 and over.

[1] Crude estimate 35.1%.

[2] Significant difference from ages 20–39.

[3] Significant difference from ages 40–59.

Figure 1. Age-adjusted prevalence of obesity, by sex and age group, among adults aged 20 and over: United States, 2011–2012.

How Many Adults Were Obese in 2011–2012?

As in 2009–2010 [3], more than 78 million adults were obese in 2011–2012. The majority of these obese adults (more than 50 million) were non-Hispanic white (Figure 3).

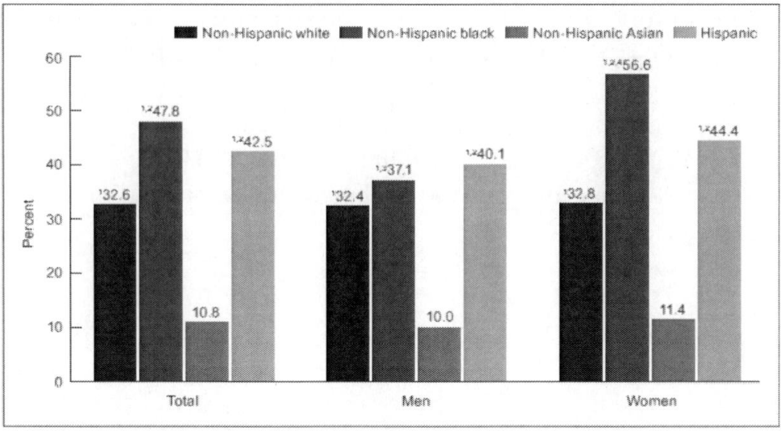

Source: CDC/NCHS, National Health and Nutrition Examination Survey, 2011–2012.

Note: Estimates are age-adjusted by the direct method to the 2000 U.S. census population using the age groups 20–39, 40–59, and 60 and over.

[1] Significant difference from non-Hispanic Asian.

[2] Significant difference from non-Hispanic white.

[3] Significant difference from women.

[4] Significant difference from Hispanic.

Figure 2. Age-adjusted prevalence of obesity, by sex and race and Hispanic origin, among adults aged 20 and over: United States, 2011–2012.

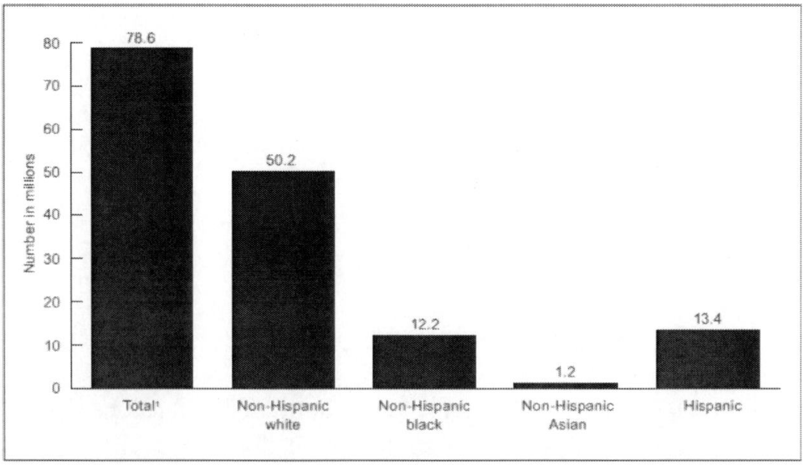

[1] Includes race and Hispanic origin groups not shown separately.

Source: CDC/NCHS, National Health and Nutrition Examination Survey, 2011–2012.

Figure 3. Number of obese adults aged 20 and over, by race and Hispanic origin: United States, 2011–2012.

DID THE PREVALENCE OF OBESITY CHANGE BETWEEN 2009–2010 AND 2011–2012?

There was no significant change in obesity prevalence between 2009–2010 and 2011–2012 among either men or women. In 2011–2012, the prevalence of obesity among men was 33.5%, compared with 35.5% in 2009–2010. Among women, obesity prevalence was 36.1% in 2011– 2012 and 35.8% in 2009–2010 (Figure 4).

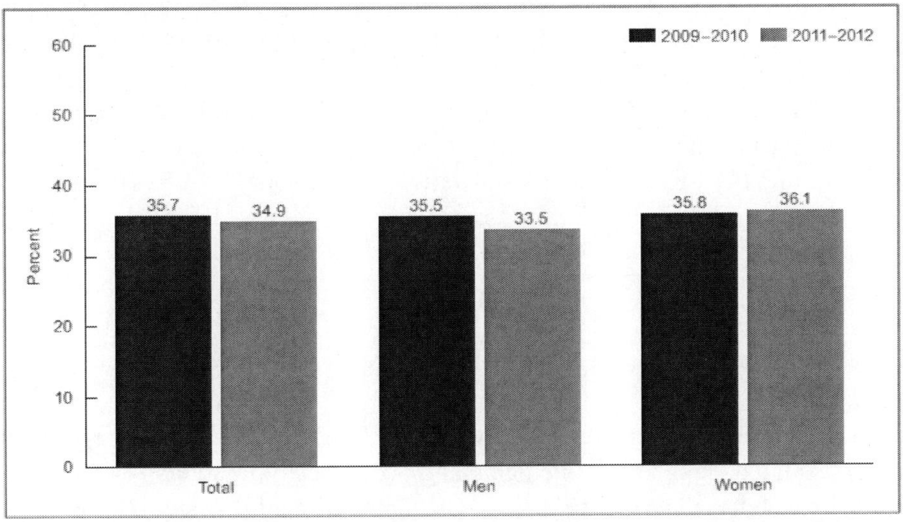

Source: CDC/NCHS, National Health and Nutrition Examination Survey, 2009–2010 and 2011–2012.

Note: Estimates are age-adjusted by the direct method to the 2000 U.S. census population using the age groups 20–39, 40–59, and 60 and over.

Figure 4. Age-adjusted prevalence of obesity, by sex, among adults aged 20 and over: United States, 2009–2010 and 2011–2012.

SUMMARY

The most recent national data from 2011–2012 on obesity prevalence among U.S. adults show that there was no significant change since 2009–2010. The prevalence of obesity among adults continues to be greater than one-third of the population.

As in 2009–2010, there was no difference in the prevalence of obesity between men and women [3]. But unlike in 2009–2010, the prevalence of obesity among the oldest adults aged 60 and over was lower, not higher, than among middle-aged adults.

Disparities in obesity prevalence continue to exist. Newly available data show a lower prevalence of obesity among non-Hispanic Asian adults than among non-Hispanic white, non-Hispanic black, and Hispanic adults. At a given body mass index (BMI) level, body fat may vary by age, sex, and racial and ethnic group [5–7]. In particular, at a given BMI, Asian adults may have more body fat than white adults [7]. Morbidity and mortality risk may be influenced by factors—such as body composition and fat distribution—that are not completely captured by BMI [8].

Disparities in obesity prevalence show the highest prevalence among non-Hispanic black and Hispanic adults. Nonetheless, the burden of obesity in terms of number of obese adults shows that the majority of obese adults are non-Hispanic white. Overall, the prevalence of obesity among U.S. adults remains above the Healthy People 2020 goal of 30.5% [9].

DEFINITION

Obesity: BMI is calculated as weight in kilograms divided by height in meters squared, rounded to one decimal place. Obesity in adults is defined as BMI greater than or equal to 30 [1]. Examples of adult obesity cut points at specific heights are shown in the Table.

Table. Obesity cut points for adults 5′4″ and 5′9″

Height	Obesity weight range
5 feet 4 inches, or 1.63 meters	174 pounds or more, or 79 kilograms or more
5 feet 9 inches, or 1.75 meters	203 pounds or more, or 92 kilograms or more

DATA SOURCE AND METHODS

Data from the National Health and Nutrition Examination Surveys (NHANES) 2011–2012 and 2009–2010 were used for these analyses. NHANES is a cross-sectional survey designed to monitor the health and nutritional status of the civilian noninstitutionalized U.S. population (10). It is conducted by the Centers for Disease Control and Prevention's (CDC) National Center for Health Statistics (NCHS). The survey consists of interviews conducted in participants' homes and standardized physical examinations conducted in mobile examination centers.

The NHANES sample is selected through a complex, multistage probability design. In 2011– 2012, non-Hispanic black, non-Hispanic Asian, and Hispanic persons, among other groups, were oversampled in order to obtain reliable estimates for these population subgroups. Race- and Hispanic origin-specific estimates reflect individuals reporting only one race; those reporting more than one race are included in the total but not reported separately.

Sample weights, which account for the differential probabilities of selection, nonresponse, and noncoverage, were incorporated into the estimation process. All variance estimates accounted for the complex survey design by using Taylor series linearization. Pregnant women were excluded from analyses.

Estimates of the number of obese adults were calculated using the alternative population control totals for 2011–2012, based on the American Community Survey [11] and on crude, rather than age-adjusted, obesity prevalence estimates.

Prevalence estimates for the total adult population were age-adjusted using the direct method to the 2000 U.S. census population using the age groups 20–39, 40–59, and 60 and over. Differences between groups were tested using a univariate t statistic at the $p < 0.05$ significance level. All differences reported are statistically significant unless otherwise indicated. Adjustments were not made for multiple comparisons. Statistical analyses were conducted using the SAS system for Windows, release 9.3 (SAS Institute Inc., Cary, N.C.) and SUDAAN, release 11.1 (RTI International, Research Triangle Park, N.C.).

About the Authors

Cynthia Ogden, Margaret Carroll, and Brian Kit are with CDC's National Center for Health Statistics, Division of Health and Nutrition Examination Surveys. Katherine Flegal is with NCHS' Office of the Director.

REFERENCES

[1] Clinical guidelines on the identification, evaluation, and treatment of overweight and obesity in adults—The evidence report. National Institutes of Health. *Obes. Res.* 6(Suppl 2):51S–209S. 1998.

[2] HHS. The surgeon general's vision for a healthy and fit nation. Rockville, MD: HHS, Office of the Surgeon General. 2010.

[3] Ogden CL, Carroll MD, Kit BK, Flegal KM. Prevalence of obesity in the United States, 2009– 2010. NCHS data brief, no 82. Hyattsville, MD: National Center for Health Statistics. 2012.

[4] Flegal KM, Carroll MD, Kit BK, Ogden CL. Prevalence of obesity and trends in the distribution of body mass index among US adults, 1999–2010. *JAMA* 307(5):491–7. 2012.

[5] Flegal KM, Ogden CL, Yanovski JA, Freedman DS, Shepherd JA, Graubard BI, Borrud LG. High adiposity and high body mass index-for-age in US children and adolescents overall and by race-ethnic group. *Am. J. Clin. Nutr.* 91(4):1020–6. 2010.

[6] Flegal KM, Shepherd JA, Looker AC, Graubard BI, Borrud LG, Ogden CL, et al. Comparisons of percentage body fat, body mass index, waist circumference, and waist-stature ratio in adults. *Am. J. Clin. Nutr.* 89(2):500–8. 2009.

[7] Deurenberg P, Deurenberg-Yap M, Guricci S. Asians are different from Caucasians and from each other in their body mass index/body fat per cent relationship. Obes Rev 3(3):141–6. 2002.

[8] Ahima RS, Lazar MA. Physiology. The health risk of obesity—Better metrics imperative. Science. 341(6148):856–8. 2013.

[9] HHS. Office of Disease Prevention and Health. Healthy People 2020 topics and objectives: Nutrition and weight status. Washington, DC. 2011. Available from: http://www.healthypeople. gov/2020/topics objectives2020/overview.aspx?topicid=29.

[10] National Center for Health Statistics. Questionnaires, datasets, and related documentation. 2012. Available from: http://www.cdc.gov/nchs/ nhanes/ nhanes_questionnaires.htm.

[11] National Center for Health Statistics. NHANES response rates and CPS totals: 2011–2012. 2013. Available from: http://www.cdc.gov/nchs/ nhanes/response_rates_CPS.htm.

INDEX

#

A

B

C

D

E

F

G

H

I

K

L

M

N

O

P

Q

R

S

T

U

V

W

Y

Z